SMOKING AND REPRODUCTION

SMOKING AND REPRODUCTION
A COMPREHENSIVE BIBLIOGRAPHY

Compiled by Ernest L. Abel

GREENWOOD PRESS
WESTPORT, CONNECTICUT • LONDON, ENGLAND

Library of Congress Cataloging in Publication Data

Abel, Ernest L., 1943-
  Smoking and reproduction.

  Includes index.
  1. Tobacco—Physiological effect—Bibliography.
2. Tobacco—Toxicology—Bibliography. 3. Fetus—Effect
of drugs on—Bibliography. 4. Generative organs—Effect
of drugs on—Bibliography. 5. Pregnant women—Tobacco
use—Bibliography. I. Title. [DNLM: 1. Fetus—Drug
effects—bibliography. 2. Smoking—In pregnancy—
Bibliography. 3. Tobacco use disorder—In pregnancy—
Bibliography. 4. Tobacco use disorder—Physiopathology—
Bibliography. 5. Nicotine—Adverse effects—Bibliography.
ZQV 137 A139s]
Z6671.2.T63A26 1982   016.61665   82-15660
[RG627.6.T6]
ISBN 0-313-23663-1 (lib bdg.)

Library of Congress Catalog Card Number: 82-15660
ISBN: 0-313-23663-1

First published in 1982

Greenwood Press
A division of Congressional Information Service, Inc.
88 Post Road West
Westport, Connecticut 06881

Printed in the United States of America

10 9 8 7 6 5 4 3 2 1

Contents

Preface

This bibliography lists various titles relating to tobacco and its effects on reproduction. As such, materials dealing with sexual behavior, sexual function, and sexual physiology have been included along with the many articles dealing with tobacco's effects on the conceptus. Most of the articles, however, have to do with the latter.

This bibliography is a comprehensive but by no means exhaustive compilation of the world literature on smoking and reproduction. Many of the citations not originally in English have been referenced as they appeared, and I have translated them or used the translation provided. In some instances, however, only the English translation is provided, because it was impossible to duplicate the original with the means available, for example, Japanese entries.

Titles are arranged alphabetically by author. An "Addendum" is also arranged in this way, and these latter entries contain items that were inadvertently omitted in the initial listing or were published after that listing. All items are numbered consecutively and are referred to by number in the subject index. The termination date for listing was May 1982.

In producing bibliographies such as this, the services and cooperation of many people are to be gratefully acknowledged. Among those to whom special appreciation is extended is Diane Augustino, librarian of the Research Institute on Alcoholism. Without Ms. Augustino's expertise many of the articles included in this volume could not have been located or verified.

Introduction

Tobacco is a flowering perennial plant. It is a member of the *Solanaceae* family which also includes henbane, deadly nightshade, and the potato. There are several different varieties of the plant, but the main one is *Nicotiana tabacum* L.

Tobacco (*Nicotiana tabacum* L.) is native to the Americas. It was first seen by Europeans during Columbus's voyage to Cuba in 1492. The word tobacco is derived from the Spanish word *taboca*, which in turn is derived from *tobago*, the Indian word for the pipe used to smoke tobacco.

Tobacco was first introduced into Europe via Spain and Portugal around 1550. In 1559, Jean Nicot,the French ambassador to Lisbon, sent some tobacco seeds to France, and in 1561 when he returned he brought some plants with him. Soon thereafter the plant became known as Nicotiana for a time.

Initially tobacco was regarded as a useful medicinal, and because of its alleged curative properties it quickly spread over Europe. Tobacco smoking for pleasure was first popularized in England by Walter Raleigh. In fact tobacco smoking became so popular in England that schools were even established to teach would-be devotees how to smoke properly. Because of the great demand for the plant, prices soared. To meet the demand and take advantage of this popularity, English colonists in the New World, especially in Virginia, began to cultivate the plant, and tobacco became a staple of the colonial economy.

The first challenge to the use of the plant was King James I's tract, "Counter-blaste to Tobacco," which denounced smoking as "a custom loathsome to the eye, hateful to the nose, harmful to the braine, (and) dangerous to the lungs . . . ."

Owing to James I's animosity to smoking, the first debate over tobacco's harmful effects was held in 1605 at Oxford University. The debate was not settled and has continued up to the present time. In other parts of the world the criticism of smoking took more violent forms than written polemics or debates. In 1634, for example, the Czar of Russia made it a crime to use tobacco. The penalty for a first offense was a whipping; for a second offense, the penalty was death!

At first tobacco was mostly smoked in pipes, but pipe smoking was soon rivaled by snuff taking. By the 1800s cigar smoking was introduced, and it challenged the pipe and snuff box for the attention of tobacco users. The cigar itself gave way to the cigarette by the 1850s. The manufacture of these "small cigars" opened up a vast new market potential, since they were much cheaper than cigars. By 1885 over one billion cigarettes had been sold in the United States. By 1888 one firm in Richmond, Virginia, was producing over two million cigarettes a day! Such mass production was brought about by the invention of the cigarette-rolling maching which was patented in 1881.

Smoking continued in popularity into the twentieth century. By 1920 the average yearly per capita consumption was about 665 cigarettes; by 1950 it was about 3,500; and by 1978 it was about 4,000.

Very few women smoked cigarettes until the 1920s. A slogan from a present-day advertisement for smoking refers to the rarity of women smoking then compared to today with the proclamation: "You've come a long way, Baby."

In the 1920s, only about 5 percent of the adult female population in the United States smoked. The percentage of women smoking has continued to increase since that time, and in the 1970s and 1980s the percentage of adult female smokers was estimated at around 30 percent. By comparison the percentage of men smoking has decreased from about 50 percent in the 1920s to about 35 to 40 percent in the 1970s and 1980s.

About 35 percent of the female population of child-bearing age smokes at the present time. Among those women who smoke, the average number of cigarettes consumed per day is about 9.5. Studies of pregnant women around the world indicate that the percentage of women smoking during pregnancy is roughly the same in all industrialized countries.

Comparisons between men and women in terms of smoking may be misleading for a number of reasons. For example, women do not smoke as much of a cigarette as men, nor do they inhale as deeply. Women also prefer lower tar and nicotine brands, so they are exposed to less tobacco and tobacco products than men even though they may smoke the same number of cigarettes.

The accuracy of surveys of smoking behavior has also been questioned. One study, for example, found that cigarette consumption based on self-reported smoking was about three-quarters of the actual cigarette sales in 1964 and about two-thirds in 1975. Estimates of smoking are thus more likely to be lower than the actual amount of smoking for individuals.

CHEMISTRY AND PHARMACOLOGY OF TOBACCO

Tobacco (*Nicotiana tabacum* L.) is cultivated in nearly every country of the world. Although primarily smoked in the form of cigarettes, cigars, or pipes, it is also chewed.

Tobacco smoke is generally divided into two main components—the gas phase and the particulate phase. The gas phase consists of smoke that passes through a specifically devised filter which screens out particles greater than 0.1 micron in diameter. The particulate phase consists of those particles which do not pass through the filter. Nicotine, one of the main components of the particulate phase of cigarette smoke, is generally regarded as the substance in tobacco responsible for reinforcing smoking, and its actions have been more widely studied than any of the more than 2,000 other compounds in tobacco.

Nicotine is a colorless to pale yellow fluid which is very soluble in water and lipids. It has a low boiling point and therefore vaporizes readily as tobacco burns during the smoking process. Nicotine is a very toxic material, and in humans the lethal dose is about forty milligrams.

As a result of its solubility, nicotine is rapidly distributed throughout all tissues and fluids of the body. Areas that achieve the highest concentrations are the brain and the pituitary and adrenal glands. In the brain nicotine is concentrated primarily in the hippocampus.

Metabolism of nicotine occurs in the liver, kidneys, and lungs. The two main metabolites are cotinine and nicotine-1-N-oxide. No metabolism occurs in the brain.

Elimination of nicotine and its metabolites from the body occurs via the kidneys. Half the amount of nicotine in the blood is removed in about forty minutes. The metabolite, cotinine, however, can still be detected in blood for several days after smoking.

Nicotine is considered a prototypic excitor of a group of neurotransmitter receptors that are called cholinergic. Nicotine depolarizes these receptors, thereby initiating nerve stimulation. This stimulation is followed by a blockade of the same receptors resulting in a decrease in nerve activity. In addition, nicotine stimulates the release of adrenaline from the adrenal glands. This results in an increase in heart rate, vasoconstriction, and oxygen consumption, among other effects which may impact adversely on a developing fetus.

Passage of nicotine across the placenta has been known since the 1930s. Both nicotine and cotinine have also been detected in amniotic fluid from pregnant women who smoked during the second trimester of gestation. Cotinine has also been found in the amniotic fluid of nonsmokers as a result of passive inhalation of cigarette smoke from other smokers. Levels were considerably below those found in the amniotic fluid of smokers, however.

It has also been known for some time that nicotine is secreted into breast milk, and there are some reports of nicotine poisoning in infants who nursed at the breast of women who were heavy smokers. While some studies have found that smoking affects milk production, this observation has not been corroborated by other studies. Women who smoke, however, have been found to stop breast feeding their children sooner than nonsmokers. Whether this is due to decreased milk production or other factors unrelated to lactation has not been studied as yet.

EFFECTS ON SEXUAL BEHAVIOR, FUNCTION, AND PHYSIOLOGY

Soon after tobacco was introduced into Europe and many Europeans began to take up the smoking habit, several polemics appeared which attacked the practice and listed various injurious effects that might be expected from such usage. One of the injurious effects often mentioned was a decrease in male fertility. Because tobacco smoke was hot and dry, it was argued, the only logical surmise was that it dried up the vital fluids of the body, including sperm. This accusation was repeated on numerous occasions and was finally the subject of several clinical reports in the twentieth century which indeed seemed to substantiate the claim that smoking did affect sperm. In most such studies, sperm motility was found to be significantly lower among smokers. When these men abstained from smoking, sperm motility increased for many. Resumption of smoking resulted once again in a decrease in sperm motility.

There is also some clinical evidence that smoking may be associated with impotency in some males. In one study, for example, two men who consulted a clinic because of erectile dysfunction were advised to stop smoking. Abstention for a few days resulted in restoration of erectile function. Physiological tests suggested that the problem may have been the result of impairment of penile blood pressure increases due to smoking.

Studies in animals of nicotine's effects on male sexual behavior and physiology have been inconclusive. Decreases in sexual activity or changes in reproductive organs, for example, have been attributed in many instances to the indirect effects of nicotine on food consumption or to drug-related general malaise.

There is virtually no information, anecdotal or otherwise, concerning tobacco's effects on female sexuality. Several studies in animals, however, have suggested that chronic exposure to cigarette smoke or nicotine can adversely affect ovarian function. Several studies have also shown that nicotine can affect the release of hormones involved in ovulation in animals. Several studies have also documented an earlier onset of menopause in women who smoke. One study, for example, found that menopause occurred at 49.4 years of age for a group of nonsmokers, at 48.0

years for women who smoked one to fourteen cigarettes per day, and at 47.6 years for women who smoked fifteen or more cigarettes a day. One of the explanations for this finding is that smoking may directly affect ovarian function.

SPONTANEOUS ABORTION

Suspicion that smoking might result in spontaneous abortion can be traced back to the seventeenth century. In 1692 one Dutch author claimed that there was no longer any doubt about the relationship. Seven years later the citizens of the Spanish city of Saragossa petitioned the Tobacco Monopoly not to build a factory in the town for fear that the tobacco odors might cause women to abort.

Recent studies have supported these early claims. A prospective epidemiological study conducted in New York State where abortion is legal matched women on the basis of age, parity, marital status, ethnicity, and socioeconomic class. Women who smoked were found to be almost twice as likely to have a spontaneous abortion as nonsmokers. The reason(s) for the increased rate of spontaneous abortions among smokers has not yet been identified, although in some cases the higher rate of abortions may be due to smoking-related damage to placentas.

BIRTHWEIGHT

By far the most common effect of smoking during pregnancy is a reduction in birthweight. One reason birthweight is often studied is that it is a rather good predictor of later development. Infants that weigh less than 2,500 grams at birth, for instance, have a much higher neonatal mortality rate than those who weigh 3,500 to 4,000 grams—the normal weight range for most infants.

The first scientific studies documenting the relationship between smoking and birthweight appeared in the late 1950s. These studies clearly showed that smoking during pregnancy was associated with lowered birthweight and demonstrated that this effect was dose-related, that is, the more a woman smoked, the greater the decrease in the weight of her baby. These studies also showed that this effect could not be accounted for in terms of other maternal characteristics such as age, parity, or prepregnancy weight.

The average reduction in birthweight associated with smoking is about 200 grams (seven ounces). Children born to mothers who smoke during pregnancy also tend to be about 1.4 centimeters shorter in length. In some studies researchers have also found a smaller head circumference among children born to smokers.

The smaller size of the infants born to smokers is due to intrauterine growth retardation rather than premature delivery, since in most studies infants of smokers are born only a few days earlier than those born to nonsmokers, and the difference in time of birth is not enough to account for the difference in size.

Also of significance is the higher incidence of "low birth weight" (2,500 grams or less) babies among smokers. Such infants have a much higher neonatal mortality rate than infants who weigh more at birth.

One explanation for the smaller size of the children born to smokers is that such women are more likely to give birth to smaller infants whether they smoke during pregnancy or not. This is called the "constitutionality hypothesis," and it contends that some physiological characteristic of the mother, rather than her smoking, is responsible for her smaller child; the fact that she smokes is incidental. However, studies comparing the weights of babies born to women who smoked during one pregnancy but not another have discredited this argument. When the weights of the two children are compared, the birthweight is generally higher when the mother did not smoke.

NEONATAL MORTALITY

In general the stillbirth rate among smokers is higher than that among nonsmokers. Maternal smoking has also been found to increase the risk of neonatal mortality for women who are already at risk because of other factors such as age, race, or low socioeconomic status.

MALFORMATIONS

The incidence of malformations of infants attributed to smoking is very low. There are reports conducted on large numbers of women, however, that have demonstrated a significant increase in the incidence of some birth defects among smokers. Cleft palate and congenital heart defects, for example, seem to occur more frequently among children born to smokers.

Studies in animals have shown that large doses of nicotine are capable of producing structural malformations in developing fetuses. When nicotine was injected into chick embryos, the embryos stopped moving within minutes of administration, suggesting depression of the brain. Spinal defects have also been produced in chicks given nicotine.

In another report an "epidemic" of limb deformities was reported in swine that had inadvertently eaten tobacco stalks.

SUDDEN INFANT DEATH SYNDROME

Several studies have reported an association between smoking and sudden infant death syndrome (also known as cot death or crib death). In one study the incidence of sudden infant death syndrome was positively related to the number of cigarettes smoked per day.

Studies in animals suggest that one reason for the association between smoking and this syndrome may be that nicotine produces lesions in that part of the developing brain that controls breathing.

LONG-TERM EFFECTS OF MATERNAL SMOKING ON OFFSPRING

In addition to its effects on spontaneous abortion, birthweight, and perinatal mortality, maternal smoking during pregnancy has been found to result in a number of adverse consequences for children long after birth.

Although not substantial, the body weights and lengths of children born to smokers are generally below those born to nonsmokers at birth and remain so as late as eleven years after birth. In some cases head circumference (an indirect measure of brain growth) is also lower among children of smokers.

Several studies have also shown that children born to smokers suffer far higher incidences of pneumonia and bronchitis than do children born to nonsmokers. Children of ex-smokers resemble nonsmokers in this regard, ruling out the possibility that children of smokers would suffer from these conditions whether their mothers smoked or not. Other studies have shown that infants born to smokers have depressed immune systems at birth. This may be one of the reasons for the higher rates of pneumonia and bronchitis for children of smokers.

Although smokers have a higher incidence of cancer than do nonsmokers, there is very little evidence that children exposed to cigarette smoke *in utero* are more likely to develop cancer later on in life. Studies in animals, on the other hand, suggest that this possibility cannot be dismissed. In one study, for example, hamsters exposed to cigarette smoke had a far higher incidence of tumors at fifteen months of age than did control animals. Fifteen months is a relatively old age for the hamster. In contrast the best human studies have not followed children exposed to cigarette smoke for longer than ten years after birth. Conceivably, extending the period of study to a later age could turn up a significant biological association between maternal smoking and cancer among children.

Several studies have begun to examine the behavioral consequences of prenatal exposure to cigarette smoke. In one such study infants born to women who smoked and drank, slept more often in an atypical head orientation to the left, appeared in a more dazed condition, yawned and sneezed more often, and were less visually alert than children born to women who smoked or drank the same amount, but did not do both. This finding suggests the possibility that while smoking may in itself not cause damage to the developing fetus, smoking may interact with other risk factors such as alcohol, to significantly alter fetal development. Other studies, however, have shown that smoking as a sole factor is capable of adversely affecting behavior of offspring.

Babies born to smokers, for example, have been found to have a weaker suck, to take longer to begin sucking, and to take longer to finish sucking, compared to other children. In another study children were evaluated at four years of age in their own homes. Those born to smokers were rated as more stubborn and persistent than other children.

In an in-depth study of 17,000 children born in England whose development was followed for several years after birth, children born to smokers lagged behind their peers in reading ability at age seven. When these children were eleven years of age their reading comprehension, mathematics, and general ability scores were below those of other children.

Other investigators have found that at six and a half years of age children born to smokers did not perform as well as other children on psychomotor tasks, in language development, or on IQ tests.

There is also some suggestive evidence that children prenatally exposed to cigarette smoke are more likely to be hyperactive when they grow older. When twenty hyperactive children were matched with twenty nonhyperactive dyslexic children and with twenty control children, the researchers found that the hyperactive children were much more likely to have been born to mothers who had smoked during pregnancy.

These observations have been duplicated to a degree in animal experiments. When rats were prenatally exposed to nicotine, for example, they were less active and did not do as well later on in learning tasks as did rats that had not been so exposed. Other experiments with animals have shown that offspring exposed to nicotine during pregnancy have significantly shorter life spans than those not exposed, and that animals exposed to nicotine or tobacco *in utero* have fewer brain cells than control animals.

EXPLANATIONS FOR THE EFFECTS OF SMOKING ON FETAL DEVELOPMENT

Although there is now no longer any doubt that smoking during pregnancy can adversely affect the developing fetus, there is still some uncertainty about the way(s) in which this damage occurs.

One interesting proposal commonly referred to as the "constitutionality hypothesis" contends that it is the woman who smokes, not the cigarette smoke, that is responsible for many of the effects associated with maternal smoking. The point of this argument is that women who smoke have some unique physiological characteristics that adversely affect their developing fetuses. The fact that they smoke is incidental.

While difficult to disprove completely, the "constitutionality hypothesis" has been weakened by numerous studies. For example, when a smoker stops smoking during pregnancy, her child resembles that of a nonsmoker much more than that of a smoker in most cases. Studies that examine successive pregnancies have also shown that the child born during the pregnancy in which the woman smoked generally weighs less than that born when the woman did not smoke. A third body of evidence against this hypothesis comes from the animal literature which has shown that animals prenatally exposed to cigarette smoke or nicotine have lower birthweights and differ in other important characteristics from nonexposed animals. Since these animals are selected at random to be exposed to cigarette smoke or nicotine, and since their life histories are tightly controlled so that the only difference between drug-treated groups and controls is the drug treatment per se, the differences between offspring cannot be attributed to unique preexisting physiological characteristics between nicotine-treated and control animals.

Somewhat related to the "constitutionality hypothesis" is the argument that the effects of smoking are indirectly mediated by smoking's effects on maternal weight gain during pregnancy. The essence of this argument is that smoking results in decreased eating and therefore reduced nutrient availability to the fetus. However, several studies have now shown that women who smoke during pregnancy gain the same amount, if not more weight than nonsmokers.

The most widely endorsed hypothesis relating maternal smoking to adverse fetal development is that smoking causes intrauterine hypoxia. Smoking-related hypoxia could occur in a number of ways, any one of which would be detrimental to development.

One way in which hypoxia from smoking could occur is by increasing the carbon monoxide in the blood. Carbon monoxide is one of the byproducts of smoking, and it has a higher affinity for hemoglobin than does oxygen. As a result carbon monoxide combines with hemoglobin to form carboxyhemoglobin. Carboxyhemoglobin levels in pregnant nonsmokers range from about 0.4 to 4.4 percent. In chronic smokers levels vary from 2 to 14 percent. The result of such increases in carboxyhemoglobin levels is a serious decrease in the oxygen-carrying capacity of the blood resulting in decreased oxygen to the fetus.

In addition to competing with oxygen for hemoglobin, carbon monoxide also decreases oxygen unloading from hemoglobin. This also has the effect of decreasing oxygen availability to the fetus.

Studies in which fetal breathing movements have been measured have demonstrated that smoking increases fetal apnea for as long as twenty seconds. In one study, fetal breathing movements dropped by about 50 percent within five minutes of smoking two cigarettes, and the level of fetal breathing did not return to presmoking levels for about one hour.

Some researchers cite comparisons between birthweights of children born at different altitudes as additional support for the hypoxia hypothesis. At higher altitudes where there is less oxygen, there is less maternal oxygen partial pressure and oxyhemoglobin than at lower altitudes. As a result, babies born at higher altitudes weigh less at birth and have higher perinatal mortality rates than those born at lower altitudes.

Another way in which smoking can cause fetal hypoxia is by reducing blood flow to the placenta. Such reductions can occur as a result of smoking-induced releases of adrenaline from the adrenal glands. Since adrenaline causes uterine vasoconstriction, this will reduce the blood flow to the placenta.

Direct effects on the placenta have also been demonstrated, and these effects could also result in decreased oxygen supply to the fetus. Smoking, for example, is associated with premature separation of the placenta from the uterine wall, suboptimal implantation of the placenta, and lesions in the placenta. Smoking also causes damage to umbilical veins and arteries.

EDUCATION AND PREVENTION

Since the late 1950s there has been increasing recognition of the harm that smoking can cause to the developing fetus. Although there have been numerous campaigns to educate the public about the deleterious effects of smoking in general, little attention is specifically devoted to the effects of smoking during pregnancy in prenatal classes. One study found that the reasons for this lack of attention are insufficient time, lack of appropriate materials, poor preparation of professionals, and a hesitancy about creating a psychological burden for the expectant mother.

Another study found that most pregnant women were aware of the social expectations concerning smoking during pregnancy, and that there was a positive correlation between such social expectations and continuation of smoking during pregnancy.

In a third study that evaluated attempts to reduce or eliminate smoking during pregnancy, researchers found that women who stopped smoking tended to be better informed about hygiene than those who did not.

In many cases women will often spontaneously reduce their use of cigarettes or will stop using them completely because of nausea or changes in taste. However, studies of preventative programs indicate that informing women about the health consequences of smoking for their developing child may give them additional incentive to reduce their smoking.

_____ Bibliography

1. Abel, E. L. Smoking during pregnancy: A review of effects on growth and development of offspring. Human Biology 1980, 52, 593-625.

2. Abel, E. L., Dintcheff, B. A. and Day, N. Effects of in utero exposure to alcohol, nicotine, and alcohol plus nicotine, on growth and development in rats. Neurobehavioral Toxicology, 1979, 1, 153-159.

3. Abernathy, J. R., Greenberg, B. G., Wells, H. B. and Frazier, T. M. Smoking as an independent variable in a multiple regression analysis upon birth weight and gestation. American Journal of Public Health and the Nation's Health, 1966, 56, 626-633.

4. Achtel, R. A. and Erickson, J. L. Left ventricular contractility in newborns of smoking mothers. Pediatric Research, 1976, 10, 327.

5. Ademowore, A. S., Courey, N. G., and Kime, J. S. Relationships of maternal nutrition and weight gain to newborn birthweight. Obstetrics and Gynecology, 1972, 39, 460-465.

6. Aeschbacher, H. U. and Chappuis, C. Non-mutagenicity of urine from coffee drinkers compared with that from cigarette smokers. Mutation Research, 1981, 89, 161-177.

7. Alberman, E. Sociobiologic factors and birth weight in Great Britain. In Reed, D. M. and Stanley, F. J. (eds.), The Epidemiology of Prematurity. Urban and Schwarzenberg, Baltimore, 1976, 145-156.

8. Alberman, E., Creasy, M., Elliott, M. and Spicer, C. Maternal factors associated with fetal chromosomal anomalies in spontaneous abortions. British Journal of Obstetrics and Gynaecology, 1976, 83, 621-627.

9.   Alberman, E., Pharoah, P. and Chamberlain, G. Smoking and
        the fetus. Lancet, 1977, 2, 36.

10.   Alpert, J. J., Day, N., Dooling, E., Hingson, R., Oppenheimer,
        E., Rosett, H. L., Weiner, L. and Zuckerman, B.
        Maternal alcohol consumption and newborn assessment:
        Methodology of the Boston City Hospital prospective
        study. Neurobehavioral Toxicology and Teratology,
        1981, 3, 195-201.

11.   Alvear, J. and Brooke, O. G. Effect of smoking on fetal
        growth. Lancet, 1977, 1, 1158.

12.   Ambache, N. and Zar, M. A. Evidence against adrenergic
        motor transmission in the guinea-pig vas deferens.
        Journal of Physiology, 1971, 216, 359-389.

13.   Amelar, R. D., Dubin, L., and Schoenfeld, C. Sperm motility.
        Fertility and Sterility, 1980, 34, 197-215.

14.   American Academy of Pediatrics Committee on Environment
        Hazards. Effects of cigarette-smoking on the fetus
        and the child. Pediatrics, 1976, 57, 411-413.

15.   Andrews, J. Thiocyanate and smoking in pregnancy.
        Journal of Obstetrics and Gynaecology, British
        Commonwealth, 1973, 80, 810-815.   ,

16.   Andrews, J. and McGarry, J. M. A community study of
        smoking in pregnancy. Journal of Obstetrics and
        Gynaecology, British Commonwealth, 1972, 79, 1057-1073.

17.   Anonymous. Smoking during pregnancy. British Medical
        Journal, 1968, 1, 339-340.

18.   Anonymous. Stillbirths and infant mortality. Medical
        Officer, 1969, 121, 116-117.

19.   Anonymous. Is smoking teratogenic? Medical Journal of
        Australia, 1971, 2, 644.

20.   Anonymous. Is tobacco teratogenic? Medical Journal of
        Australia, 1972, 18, 896.

21.   Anonymous. El habito de fumar y las enfermedades. 1.
        (The smoking habit and the infirmities). Prensa
        Medica Mexicana, 1972, 37, 351-353.

22.   Anonymous. Reflections for smoking mothers. Food and
        Cosmetics Toxicology, 1973, 1, 671-674.

23.   Anonymous. Smoking and pregnancy. Medical Journal of
        Australia, 1973, 1, 671.

24.   Anonymous. Smoking and pregnancy. Nature, 1973, 246,
        177-178.

25.   Anonymous. Smoking hazard to the fetus. British Medical
       Journal, 1973, 1, 369-370.

26.   Anonymous. Smoking, pregnancy, and development of the
       offspring. Nutrition Reviews, 1973, 31, 143-145.

27.   Anonymous. Smoking, pregnancy and publicity. Nature,
       1973, 245, 467-468.

28.   Anonymous. Smoking in pregnancy and child development.
       British Medical Journal, 1974, 1, 610-611.

29.   Anonymous. Effects of cigarette-smoking on the fetus
       and child. Pediatrics, 1976, 57, 411-413.

30.   Anonymous. Is tobacco teratogenic? Medical Journal of
       Australia, 1977, 1, 896.

31.   Anonymous. Smoking during pregnancy. American Lung
       Association Bulletin, 1977, 63, 9.

32.   Anonymous. In smoke-filled wombs, trouble looms.
       Medical World News, 1977, August 22, 7.

33.   Anonymous. Da hilft nur Verzicht auf Alkohol und Zigar-
       etten: Schwangere Gefährden ihr King-Wissenschaftliche
       Studie über "Schwangerschaftsverlauf und Kindesenticklung".
       (So only renunciation of alcohol and cigarettes helps:
       Pregnancy risks to her in King's scientific study on
       "Course of pregnancy and child development".)
       Schwestern Revue, 1977, 15, 11-12.

34.   Anonymous. Smoking and pregnancy. South African Medical
       Journal, 1977, 2, 1106-1107.

35.   Anonymous. Smoking and the fetus. Lancet, 1977, 2,
       36-37.

36.   Anonymous. Tobacco may cause placental separation.
       Medical World News, 1977, May 2, 33-34.

37.   Anonymous. Cigarette smoking and spontaneous abortion.
       British Medical Journal, 1978, 1, 259.

38.   Anonymous. Placental defects linked to smoking.
       Medical World News, 1978, November 27, 25-26.

39.   Anonymous. Smoking, Drinking, and Pregnancy. Do It Now
       Foundation Institute for Chemical Survival, Phoenix,
       Arizona, 1978.

40.   Anonymous. Dangers of smoking during pregnancy reported.
       American Family Physician, 1980, 21, 203-206.

41.   Anonymous. Mothers who smoke and their children. Report
       of Committee appointed by Action on Smoking and Health.
       Practitioner, 1980, 224, 735-740.

42.   Anonymous. Hazards of tobacco smoking in human reproduction.
       Pediatrics, 1980, 65, 250.

43.   Ashton, H. Cigarette smoking in pregnancy: Differences
       in peripheral circulation between smokers and non-
       smokers. British Journal of Obstetrics and Gynaecology,
       1975, 82, 868-881.

44.   Ashton, H. Effect of smoking on carboxyhaemoglobin
       level in pregnancy. British Medical Journal, 1976,
       1, 42-43.

45.   Asmussen, I. Arterial changes in infants of smoking
       mothers. Postgraduate Medical Journal, 1978, 54,
       200-204.

46.   Asmussen, I. Ultrastructure of human umbilical veins:
       Observations of veins from newborn children of smoking
       and nonsmoking mothers. Acta Obstetrica et Gynecologica
       Scandinavica, 1978, 57, 253-255.

47.   Asmussen, I. Fetal cardiovascular system as influenced
       by maternal smoking. Clinical Cardiology, 1979, 2,
       246-256.

48.   Asmussen, I. Tobacco smoking during pregnancy--Clinical
       implications for the next generation. Danish Medical
       Bulletin, 1980, 27, 118.

49.   Asmussen, I. and Kjeldsen, K. Intimal ultrastructure of
       human umbilical arteries. Observations on arteries
       from newborn children of smoking and nonsmoking mothers.
       Circulation Research, 1975, 36, 579-581.

50.   Astrup, P. Carbon monoxide in tobacco smoke and its
       influence on the development of vascular diseases.
       Rehabilitation, 1972, 25, 11-12.

51.   Astrup, P., Olsen, H. M., Trolle, D. and Kjeldsen, K.
       Effect of moderate carbon-monoxide exposure on fetal
       development. Lancet, 1972, 2, 1221-1222.

52.   Auerbach, O. Changes in the bronchial epithelium in
       relation to smoking and cancer of the lung. New
       England Journal of Medicine, 1957, 256, 97-104.

53.   Avendano, O. El habito de fumar y su influencia en
       el proceso de la reproduccion humana. (The smoking
       habit and its influence on the process of human
       reproduction.) Revista Chilena de Obstetrica y
       Ginecologia, 1974, 39, 119-120.

B

54.   Baer, D. S., McClearn, G. E. and Wilson, J. R. Fertility
      maternal care, and offspring behavior in mice prenatally
      treated with tobacco smoke. Developmental Psycho-
      biology, 1980, 13, 643-652.

55.   Bailey, A., Robinson, D., and Vessey, M. Smoking and
      age of natural menopause. Lancet, 1977, 2, 722.

56.   Bailey, R. R. The effect of maternal smoking on the infant
      birth weight. New Zealand Medical Journal, 1970,
      71, 293-294.

57.   Banyai, A. L. Smoking. Some of its less publicized
      sequels. Chest, 1976, 69, 55.

58.   Baric, L. and MacArthur, C. Health norms in pregnancy.
      British Journal of Preventive and Social Medicine,
      1977, 31, 30-38.

59.   Baric, L., MacArthur, C. and Sherwood, M. A study of
      health education aspects of smoking in pregnancy.
      International Journal of Health Education, 1976,
      19, 1-15.

60.   Barnes, D. E., King, M. A., Goldberg, D. and Harris, J. A.
      Effect of prenatal exposure to cigarette smoke on
      rat neurogenesis. Teratology, 1981, 23, 25A-26A.

61.   Barnwell, S. L. and Sastry, B. V. R. Influence of nicotine
      and tobacco gases on the uptake of neutral amino
      acids by isolated human placental villus. Toxicology
      and Applied Pharmacology, 1979, 48, A117.

62.   Becker, R. F. and King, J. E. Studies on nicotine
      absorption during pregnancy. II. The effects of acute
      heavy doses on mother and neonates. American Journal
      of Obstetrics and Gynecology, 1966, 95, 515-522.

63.   Becker, R. F., Little, C. R. D. and King, J. E. Exper-
       imental studies on nicotine absorption in rats during
       pregnancy. III. Effect of subcutaneous injection of
       small chronic doses upon mother, fetus and neonate.
       American Journal of Obstetrics and Gynecology, 1968,
       100, 957-968.

64.   Becker, R. F. and Martin, J. C. Vital effects of chronic
       nicotine absorption and chronic hypoxic stress
       during pregnancy and the nursing period. American
       Journal of Obstetrics and Gynecology, 1971, 110,
       522-533.

65.   Behrend, A. and Thienes, C. H. Failure of nicotine to
       alter estrus cycle in white rat. Proceedings of the
       Society for Experimental Biology and Medicine,
       1931, 28, 740-741.

66.   Behrend, A. and Thienes, C. H. Chronic nicotinism in
       young rats and rabbits. Effect on growth and estrus.
       Journal of Pharmacology and Experimental Therapeutics,
       1932, 46, 113-124.

67.   Behrend, A. and Thienes, C. H. The development of tolerance
       to nicotine by rats. Journal of Pharmacology and
       Experimental Therapeutics, 1933, 48, 317-325.

68.   Benigni, P. F. Sulle alterazioni anatomiche indotte
       dall'intossicazione cronica sperimentale da tabacco.
       (Anatomical changes induced by chronic experimental
       intoxication with tobacco.) Revista di Patologia
       Nervosa, 1911, 16, 80-100.

69.   Benz, J. Female infertility. Praxis, 1980, 69, 1769-
       1773.

70.   Bergman, A. B., Beckwith, J. B. and Ray, C. (eds.).
       Sudden Infant Death Syndrome: Proceedings of the
       Second International Conference of Causes of Sudden
       Death in Infants. University of Washington Press,
       Seattle, 1970.

71.   Bergman, A. B. and Wiesner, L. A. Relationship of passive
       cigarette smoking to sudden infant death syndrome.
       Pediatrics, 1976, 58, 665-668.

72.   Berke, R. Prenatal Exposure to Cigarette Smoke: Effects
       on Rat Offspring Behavior. Ph.D. Thesis, Yeshiva
       University, 1973.

73.   Bernhard, P. Der Einfluss des Zigarettenrauchens auf die
       schwangere Frau. (The influence of cigarette
       smoking on the pregnant woman.) Zentralblatt für
       Gynäkologie, 1948, 70, 18-30.

74.   Bernhard, P. Die Wirkung des Rauchens auf Frau und
       Mutter. (The effects of smoking in women and
       mothers.) Münchener Medizinische Wochenschrift,
       1962, 104, 1826-1831.

75.   Berry, E. M. Sperm abnormalities and cigarette smoking.
       Lancet, 1981, 1, 1159.

76.   Betz, E. H. Le tabagisme et ses dangers. (Tobacco use and
       its dangers.) Revue Médicale, 1972, 27, 615-618.

77.   Bisdom, C. J. W. Alcohol en nicotinever giftigung bij
       zuigelinger. (Alcohol and nicotine poisoning in
       infants.) Maandscrift voor Kindergeneeskunde,
       1937, 6, 332-341.

78.   Bisset, G. W. and Walker, J. M. The effects of nicotine,
       hexamethonium, and ethanol on the secretion of the
       anti-diuretic and oxytocic hormones of the rat.
       British Journal of Pharmacology, 1957, 12, 461-467.

79.   Biswas, N. M., Paul, B., and Sarkar, D. Role of phentol-
       amine on the length of pregnancy and fetal development
       in nicotine-treated pregnant rats. Endokrinologie,
       1977, 69, 359-360.

80.   Blake, C. A. Parallelism and divergence in LH and FSH
       release in nicotine-treated rats. Proceedings of
       the Society for Experimental Biology and Medicine,
       1974, 145, 706-710.

81.   Blake, C. A. Paradoxical effects of drugs acting on the
       central nervous system on the preovulatory release of
       pituitary luteinizing hormone in proestrous rats.
       Journal of Endocrinology, 1978, 79, 319-326.

82.   Blake, C. A., Norman, R. L., Scaramuzzi, R. J. and
       Sawyer, C. H. Inhibition of the proestrous surge of
       prolactin in the rat by nicotine. Endocrinology,
       1973, 91, 1334-1338.

83.   Blake, C. A. and Sawyer, C. H. Nicotine blocks the
       suckling-induced rise in circulating prolactin in
       lactating rats. Science, 1972, 177, 619-621.

84.   Blake, C. A., Scaramuzzi, R. J., Norman, R. L., Kanematsu, S.,
       and Sawyer, C. H. Effect of nicotine on the proestrus
       ovulatory surge of LH in the rat. Endocrinology,
       1972, 91, 1253-1258.

85.   Blake, C. A., Scaramuzzi, R. J., Norman, R. L., Kanematsu, S.,
       and Sawyer, C. H. Nicotine delays the ovulatory surge
       of luteinizing hormone in the rat. Proceedings of the
       Society for Experimental Biology, 1972, 141, 1014-1016.

86.   Blakey, D. Smoking mothers and infant health. Journal
       of the Mississippi State Medical Association, 1975,
       16, 14.

87.   Bosley, A. R., Newcome, R. G. and Dauncey, M. E. Maternal
       smoking and Apgar score. Lancet, 1981, 1, 337-338.

88.   Boué, J., Boué, A., and Lazar, P. Retrospective and
       prospective epidemiological studies of 1500 karyo-
       typed spontaneous human abortions. Teratology,
       1975, 12, 11-26.

89.   Boyce, A., Schwartz, D., Hubert, C., Cedara, L. and
       Dreyfus, J. Smoking, human placental lactogen and
       birth weight. British Journal of Obstetrics and Gyne-
       cology, 1976, 82, 964-967.

90.   Branch, H. E. and Moss, W. G. Effects of nicotine on
       rats (albino). Transactions of the Kansas Academy
       of Sciences, 1938, 41, 317-329.

91.   Breen, H., Demarsico, R. and Gregori, C. A. Smoking
       and pregnancy. Journal of the Medical Society of
       New Jersey, 1978, 75, 124-135.

92.   Bresch, H., Spielhoff, R. and Mohr, U. Use of the sea
       urchin egg for quick screen testing of the biological
       activities of substances. I. Influence of fractions
       of a tobacco smoke condensate on early development.
       Proceedings of the Society for Experimental Biology
       and Medicine, 1972, 141, 747-752.

93.   Bridges, B. A., Chelmmesen, J., and Sugimura, T.
       Cigarette smoking--does it carry a genetic risk?
       Mutation Research, 1979, 65, 71-81.

94.   Briggs, M. H. Cigarette smoking and infertility in men.
       Medical Journal of Australia, 1973, 7, 616-617.

95.   Bruce, N. and Parkinson, S. Effect of nicotine on
       uterine blood flow in anesthetized pregnant rats.
       Biology of Reproduction, 1979, 21, 229-233.

96.   Buel, F., Buel, W., Fielding, F., Little, D., Little, M.
       and Thienes, C. H. Estrus and reproduction in the
       white rat as influenced by chronic nicotinism.
       Journal of Pharmacology and Experimental Therapeutics,
       (Proceedings), 1937, 60, 100.

97.   Bulay, O. M. and Wattenberg, L. W. Carcinogenic effects
       of subcutaneous administration of benzo(a)pyrene
       during pregnancy on the progeny. Proceedings of the
       Society for Experimental Biology and Medicine, 1970,
       135, 84-86.

98.   Bulzoni, S., Tecca, E., and Ilari, M. Le Intossicazioni
        Croniche in Gravidanza: da Tabagismo e da Farmaci.
        (Chronic poisoning in pregnancy: Tobacco and drugs.)
        Gassetta Internazionale Di Medicina e Chirurgia,
        1968, 73, 4710-4715.

99.   Buncher, C. R. Cigarette smoking and duration of
        pregnancy. American Journal of Obstetrics and
        Gynecology, 1969, 103, 942-946.

100.   Burch, P. R. Smoking, pregnancy and publicity. Nature,
        1973, 245, 277.

101.   Burch, P. R. Effects of cigarette smoking on the fetus
        and child. Pediatrics, 1977, 60, 766-767.

102.   Burch, P. R. Dose-response effect of maternal smoking:
        Dr. Burch replies. Pediatrics, 1978, 62, 862-863.

103.   Burch, P. R. Cancer risk from transplacental exposure
        to maternal smoking. Lancet, 1980, 2, 311.

104.   Burns, B. and Gurtner, G. H. A specific carrier for
        oxygen and carbon monoxide in the lung and placenta.
        Drug Metabolism and Disposition, 1973, 1, 374-379.

105.   Butler, N. R. The problem of low birthweight and early
        delivery. Journal of Obstetrics and Gynecology of
        the British Commonwealth, 1965, 72, 1001-1003.

106.   Butler, N. R. Risk factors in human intrauterine growth
        retardation. CIBA Foundation Symposium, 1974, 27,
        379-382.

107.   Butler, N. R. and Alberman, E. D. (eds.). Perinatal
        Problems--The Second Report of the 1958 British
        Perinatal Mortality Survey. E. & S. Livingstone Ltd.,
        Edinburgh, 1969.

108.   Butler, N. R. and Goldstein, H. Smoking in pregnancy
        and subsequent child development. British Medical
        Journal, 1973, 4, 573-575.

109.   Butler, N. R., Goldstein, H. and Ross, E. M. Cigarette
        smoking in pregnancy: Its influence on birth weight
        and perinatal mortality. British Medical Journal,
        1972, 1, 127-130.

C

110. Cameron, P., Kostin, J. S., Zaks, J. M., Wolfe, J. H.,
      Tighe, G., Oselett, B., Stocker, R. and Winton, J.
      The health of smokers' and nonsmokers' children.
      Journal of Allergy, 1969, 43, 336-340.

111. Camerson, P. and Robertson, D. Effect of home environment
      tobacco smoke on family health. Journal of Applied
      Psychology, 1973, 57, 142-147.

112. Camerson, S. J., Bain, H. H. and Grant, W. B. Ventilatory
      function in pregnancy. Scotland Medical Journal,
      1970, 15, 243-247.

113. Campbell, A. M. Excessive cigarette smoking in women and
      its effect upon their reproductive efficiency.
      Journal of the Michigan Medical Society, 1935, 34,
      146-151.

114. Campbell, A. M. The effect of excessive cigarette
      smoking on maternal health. American Journal of
      Obstetrics and Gynecology, 1936, 31, 502-508.

115. Campbell, J. M. and Harrison, K. L. Smoking and infertility.
      Medical Journal of Australia, 1979, 1, 342-343.

116. Campagnoli, C., Prelato, L., and Rossetti, M. G.
      Estrogen therapy for the climateric and thromboembolic
      risk. Minerva Ginecologia, 1980, 32, 429-435.

117. Card, J. P. and Mitchell, J. A. The effects of nicotine
      administration on deciduoma induction in the rat.
      Biology of Reproduction, 1978, 19, 326-331.

118. Card, J. P. and Mitchell, J. A. Effects of nicotine on
      implantation in the rat. Biology of Reproduction,
      1979, 20, 532-539.

119.   Carney, R. E. Sex chromatin, body masculinity, achievement
        motivation and smoking behavior. Psychological
        Reports, 1967, 20, 859-866.

120.   Caro, C. G. Umbilical arteries in smoking and nonsmoking
        mothers. Circulation Research, 1975, 37, 521.

121.   Carruth, B. R. Influence of smoking and food intake on
        weight gain of pregnant adolescents. Journal of
        Adolescent Health Care, 1980, 1, 86-91.

121a.   Cater, J. I. Correlates of low birth weight. Child Care
        Health and Development, 1980, 6, 267-277.

122.   Cederlof, R., Friberg, L. and Lundman, T. The interaction
        of smoking, environment and heredity, and their
        implications for disease etiology. Acta Medica
        Scandinavica (Supplement), 1977, 712, 1-20.

123.   Cendron, H. and Vallery-Masson, J. Tobacco and male
        sexual behavior. Vie Médicale, 1971, 25, 3027-3029.

124.   Chakraborti, A. K., Samantaray, S. K., and Johnson, S.C.
        Smoking in health and disease. Journal of the
        Indian Medical Association, 1977, 68, 84-88.

125.   Chamberlain, G. Aetiology of gynaecological cancer.
        Journal of the Royal Society of Medicine, 1981,
        74, 246-261.

126.   Chamorro, G., Lerdo De Tejada, A., Carreno, M., Berdeja, B.M.,
        and Karchmer, S. Relation between resorption and
        placental 5-hydroxytryptamine and 5-hydroxyindole-3-
        acetic acid concentrations in the rat. Ginecologia y
        Obstetrica Mexicana, 1978, 43, 211-217.

127.   Christianson, R. E. Gross differences observed in the
        placentas of smokers and nonsmokers. American
        Journal of Epidemiology, 1979, 110, 178-187.

128.   Cloeren, S. E., Lippert, T. H. and Fridrich, R. The
        influence of cigarette smoking on fetal heart rate
        and uteroplacental blood volume. Archiv fuer
        Gynaekologie, 1974, 216, 15-22.

129.   Cohlan, S. Q. Drugs and pregnancy. Progress in Clinical
        and Biological Research, 1980, 44, 77-96.

130.   Cole, P. V., Hawkins, L. H. and Roberts, D. Smoking
        during pregnancy and its effect on the fetus.
        Journal of Obstetrics and Gynecology of the British
        Commonwealth, 1972, 79, 782-787.

131.   Coleman, S., Piotrow, P. T., and Rinehart, W. Tobacco:
        Hazards to Health and Human Reproduction. Population
        Reports, Series L. Johns Hopkins University Population
        Information Program, Baltimore, 1979.

132.   Colley, J. Passive smoking in children. Nursing Times,
        1975, 71, 1858-1859.

133.   Colley, J. R. T. Respiratory symptoms in children and
        parental smoking and phlegm production. British
        Medical Journal, 1974, 2, 201-204.

134.   Colley, J. R. T., Holland, W. W., and Corkhill, R. T.
        Influence of passive smoking and parental phlegm
        on pneumonia and bronchitis in early childhood.
        Lancet, 1974, 2, 1031-1034.

135.   Comber, R. and Grasso, P. The effects of chemical
        irritants and tobacco smoke condensate on the chorio-
        allantoic membrane of the fertile hen's egg.
        Chemico--Biological Interactions, 1973, 6, 25-34.

136.   Committee on Environmental Hazards. Effects of cigarette-
        smoking on fetus and child. Pediatrics, 1976, 57,
        411-413.

137.   Comstock, G. W. and Lundin, F. E. Parental smoking and
        perinatal mortality. American Journal of Obstetrics
        and Gynecology, 1967, 98, 708-718.

138.   Comstock, G. W., Shah, F. K., Meyer, M. B. and Abbey, H.
        Low birth weight and neonatal mortality rate related
        to maternal smoking and socioeconomic status.
        American Journal of Obstetrics and Gynecology, 1971,
        111, 53-59.

139.   Condie, R. G. and Pirani, B. B. The influence of smoking
        on the haemostatic mechanism in pregnancy. Acta
        Obstetrica and Gynecologica Scandinavica, 1977,
        56, 5-8.

140.   Conney, A. H., Welch, R. and Kuntzman, R. Effects of
        environmental chemicals on the metabolism of drugs,
        carcinogens, and normal body constituents in man.
        Annals of the New York Academy of Sciences, 1971,
        179, 155-172.

141.   Cope, I., Lancaster, P. and Stevens, L. Smoking in
        pregnancy. Medical Journal of Australia, 1973, 1,
        673-677.

142.   Cope, I., Stevens, L., Lancaster, P., Sutherland, R., and
        Skilsey, S. Smoking and pregnancy. Medical Journal of
        Australia, 1975, 2, 745-747.

143.   Cotaescu, I., Deutsch, G., and Dreichlinger, O. The
        influence of caffeine, nicotine and ethanol on rat
        placentary blood circulation established by means of
        Rb^{86} uptake. Revue Roumaine d'Embryologie et de
        Cytologie (Series D, Embryologie), 2, 31-35.

144.   Coudray, P. Tobacco and female sexual behavior. Vie
        Medicale, 1971, 25, 3031-3052.

145.   Crockett, E. J. How to help the pregnant patient who
        smokes. Female Patient, 1977, 2, 4.

146.   Crowe, M. Skeletal anomalies in pigs associated with
        tobacco. Modern Veterinary Practice, 1969, 50,
        54-55.

147.   Crowe, M. Study of the teratogenic capability of tobacco
        (Nicotiana tobaccum) and those chemicals commonly
        applied to the growing plants. Tobacco Health
        Workshop Conference Proceedings, 1972, 3, 256-266.

148.   Crowe, M. Study of the teratogenic capability of tobacco
        (Nicotiana tobacum) and those chemicals commonly
        applied to the growing plant. Tobacco Health
        Workshop Conference Proceedings, 1973, 4, 198-202.

149.   Crowe, M. and Pike, H. T. Congenital arthrogryposis
        associated with ingestion of tobacco stalks by
        pregnant sows. Journal of the American Veterinary
        Association, 1973, 162, 453-455.

150.   Crowe, M. and Swerczek, T. W. Congenital arthrogryposis
        in offspring of sows fed tobacco (Nicotiana tobaccum).
        American Journal of Veterinary Research, 1974, 35,
        1071-1073.

151.   Cushny, A. R. On the movements of the uterus. Journal
        of Physiology, 1906-1907, 35, 1-19.

D

152.   Dadak, C. H., Leithner, C. H., Sinzinger, H., and
        Silberbauer, K. Diminished prostacyclin formation in
        umbilical arteries of babies born to women who
        smoke. Lancet, 1981, 1, 94.

153.   Dahlmamn, T. In-vivo and in-vitro ciliotoxic effects of
        tobacco smoke. Archives of Environmental Health,
        1970, 21, 633.

154.   Dalby, J. T. Environmental effects on prenatal development.
        Journal of Pediatric Psychology, 1978, 3, 105-109.

155.   Dale, H. H. and Laidlaw, P. P. The significance of the
        supra-renal capsules in the action of certain
        alkaloids. Journal of Physiology, 1912, 45, 1-26.

156.   Damon, A., Nuttal, R. L., Salber, E. J., Seltzer, C. C.,
        and MacMahon, B. Tobacco smoke as a possible genetic
        mutagen: Parental smoking and sex of children.
        American Journal of Epidemiology, 1966, 83, 530-536.

157.   Danaher, B. G. Obstetric and gynecology intervention in
        helping smokers quit. Paper presented at the
        International Conference on Smoking Cessation,
        New York, June 22, 1978.

158.   Danaher, B. G., Shisslak, C. M., Thompson, C. B., and
        Ford, J. D. A smoking cessation program for
        pregnant women: An exploratory study. American
        Journal of Public Health, 1978, 68, 896-898.

159.   Daniel, C., Nitzescu, I. I., Soimaru, A., and Georescu, I. D.
        Recherches experimentales sur la motilité de la
        trompe uterine de la femme. (Experimental studies
        on the motility of the female uterus). Comptes
        Rendu des Sciences de la Société de Biologie, 1935,
        120, 54-56.

160.   Daniell, H. W. Osteoporosis of the slender smoker.
        Archives of Internal Medicine, 1976, 136, 298-304.

161.   Daniell, H. W. Smoking, obesity, and the menopause.
        Lancet, 1978, 2, 373.

162.   Datey, K. K. and Dalvi, C. P. Tobacco and health.
        Indian Journal of Chest Diseases, 1972, 14, 158-167.

163.   Davie, R., Butler, N. R., and Goldstein, H. (editors).
        From Birth to Seven. Longmans, London, 1972.

164.   Davies, D. P., Gray, O. P., Ellwood, P. C., and Aber-
        nethy, M. Cigarette smoking in pregnancy: Associ-
        ations with maternal weight gain and fetal growth.
        Lancet, 1976, 1, 385-387.

165.   Davies, P. and Kister, G. S. The assessment of tobacco
        smoke toxicity in organ culture. II. Ultrastructural
        studies on the immediate response of foetal rabbit
        tracheal epithelium to short-term exposure of whole
        smoke. Experientia, 1975, 3, 682-684.

166.   Deblay, M. F. Effects nocifs du tabac pour le foetus et
        le nouveau-né. (Noxious effects of tobacco on the
        foetus and n-wborn.) Soins, 1980, 25, 19-25.

167.   Degenhardt, H. H. and Seitner, C. A. Rauchen und
        Schwangerschaft. (Smoking and pregnancy.) Med-
        izinische Klinik, 1976, 7, 1923-1927.

168.   De Haas, J. H. Parental smoking: Its effects on fetus
        and child health. European Journal of Obstetrics,
        Gynecology, and Reproductive Biology, 1975, 5, 283-
        296.

169.   Deibel, P. Effects of cigarette smoking on maternal
        nutrition and the fetus. Journal of Obstetric and
        Gynecological Nursing, 1980, 9, 333-336.

170.   DeMarsico, R., Gregori, C. A., and Breen, J. L. Smoking
        and pregnancy. Journal of the Medical Society of
        New Jersey, 1978, 75, 124-135.

171.   Denson, R., Nanson, J. L., and McWalters, M. A.
        Hyperkinesis and maternal smoking. Canadian Psy-
        chiatric Association Journal, 1975, 20, 183-187.

172.   De Zilwa, L. A. E. Some contributions to the physiology
        of unstriated muscle. Journal of Physiology, 1901-
        1902, 27, 200-223.

173.   Di Carlo, F. J. and Gilani, S. H. Disposition of 14C-
        nicotine in the fertilized chich egg. American Jour-
        nal of Anatomy, 1977, 148, 527-534.

174.   Di Carlo, F. J. and Gilani, S. H.   Effects of nicotine
        on chick embryo heart. Anatomical Record, 1977,
        187, 566.

175.   Dickens, G. and Trethowan, W. H.   Cravings and aversions
        during pregnancy. Journal of Psychosomatic Research,
        1971, 15, 259-268.

176.   Di Paolo, J. A.   Teratogenic agents: Mammalian test
        systems and chemicals. Annals of the New York
        Academy of Sciences, 1969, 163, 801-812.

177.   Divers, W. A., Wilkes, M. M., Babaknia, A., and Yen, S. S. C.
        Maternal smoking and elevation of catecholamines and
        metabolites in the amniotic fluid. American Journal
        of Obstetrics and Gynecology, 1981, 141, 625-628.

178.   Doerfel, G.   Die Wirkung des Rauchens in der Schwanger-
        schaft auf die Herzfreqenz des Feten. (The effects
        of smoking in pregnancy and on fetal heart rate.)
        Zeitschrift für die Gesamte Innere Medizin und
        Grenzgebiete, 1952, 7, 227-229.

179.   Domagala, J. and Domagala, L.   Zachowanie sie wagi
        urodzeniowej oraz czestość wystepowania wcześniactwa
        i wad wrodzonych u noworodków kobiet palacych tytoń.
        (Birth weight and incidence of prematurity and
        congenital anomalies in newborns of mothers smoking
        tobacco.)   Pediatria Polska, 1972, 47, 735-738.

180.   Donovan, J. W.   Effect on child of maternal smoking
        during pregnancy. Lancet, 1973, 1, 376.

181.   Donovan, J. W.   Randomised controlled trial of anti-
        smoking advice in pregnancy. British Journal of
        Preventive and Social Medicine, 1977, 31, 6-12.

182.   Donovan, J. W., Burgess, P. I., and Hossack, C. M.
        Routine advice against smoking in pregnancy.
        Journal of the Royal College of General Practitioners,
        1975, 25, 264-268.

183.   Dontenwill, W., Chevalier, H.-J., Harke, H.-P., Lafrenz, U.,
        Reckzeh, G., and Schneider, B.   Experimental investi-
        gations of the effect of cigarette smoke exposure on
        testicular function of Syrian golden hamsters. Tox-
        icology, 1973, 1, 309-320.

184.   Dow, T. G. B., Rooney, P. J. and Spence, M.   Does
        anemia increase the risks to the fetus caused by
        smoking in pregnancy? British Medical Journal,
        1975, 4, 253-254.

185.   Downing, G. C. and Chapman, W. E.   Smoking and pregnancy:
        A statistical study of 5,659 patients. California
        Medicine, 1966, 104, 187-191.

186.   Drac, P. and Kopecny, J. Sterility in female smokers and
        nonsmokers. Zentralblatt für Gynäkologie, 1970, 92,
        865-866.

187.   Drysdale, C. R. Tobacco, and its effects on the health
        of males. British Medical Journal, 1875, 2, 271.

188.   D'Souza, S. W., Black, P. M., Williams, N., and Jennison,
        R. F. Effect of smoking during pregnancy upon the
        haematological values of cord blood. British Journal
        of Obstetrics and Gynecology, 1978, 85, 495-499.

189.   Duffus, G. M. and MacGillivray, I. The incidence of pre-
        eclamptic toxemia in smokers and nonsmokers. Lancet,
        1968, 1, 994-995.

189a.   Dubois, J. Les grossesses à risque. (Pregnancies at
        risk.) Concours Médical, 1976, 98, 3307-3313.

190.   Dumont, N. Hypotrophie foetale et intoxications mater-
        nelles chroniques. (Intrauterine growth retardation
        and chronic maternal intoxications.) Revue Française
        de Gynécologie et d'Obstétrique, 1977, 72, 797-803.

191.   Dunachie, J. F. and Fletcher, W. W. Effect of some in-
        secticides on the hatching rate of hens' eggs. Nature,
        1966, 212, 1062-1063.

192.   Dunn, H. G. and McBurney, A. K. Cigarette smoking and the
        fetus and child. Pediatrics, 1977, 60, 772.

193.   Dunn, H. G., McBurney, A. K., Ingram, S., and Hunter, C. M.
        Maternal cigarette smoking during pregnancy and the
        child's subsequent development. 1. Physical growth to
        the age of 6½ years. Canadian Journal of Public
        Health, 1976, 67, 499-505.

194.   Dunn, H. G., McBurney, A. K., and Sandraingram, A. Mater-
        nal cigarette smoking during pregnancy and the child's
        subsequent development. II. Neurological and intel-
        lectual maturation to the age of 6½ years. Canadian
        Journal of Public Health, 1977, 68, 43-50.

195.   Dunwoody, J. Smoking. Community Health, 1973, 4, 321-
        325.

E

196.   Editorial. Smoking hazard to the fetus. British Medical
        Journal, 1973, 1, 369-370.

197.   Editorial. Smoking, pregnancy and development of the off-
        spring. Nutrition Review, 1973, 31, 143-149.

198.   Editorial. Smoking, pregnancy and publicity. Nature,
        1973, 245, 61.

199.   Editorial. A special responsibility? Nursing Times,
        1974, 70, 407.

200.   Editorial. Tobacco smoke and the non-smoker. Lancet,
        1974, 1, 1201-1202.

201.   Editorial. Cigarette smoking in pregnancy. British
        Medical Journal, 1976, 2, 492.

202.   Editorial. Smoking and pregnancy. South African Medical
        Journal, 1977, 52, 1106-1107.

203.   Edmunds, C. W. The point of attack of certain drugs
        acting on the retractor penis muscle of the dog.
        Journal of Pharmacology and Experimental Therapeutics,
        1920, 15, 201-216.

204.   Elis, J. and Kršiak, M. The effect of nicotine adminis-
        tration during pregnancy on the postnatal development
        of offspring. Acta Nervosa Superior, 1973, 15,
        148.

205.   Elliott, J. Maternal smoking and the fetus: One fear
        buried but others arise. Journal of the American
        Medical Association, 1979, 241, 867-868.

206.   Emanuel, W. Über das Vorkommen von Nicotin in der Frauen-
        milch nach Zigarettengenuss. (On the presence of nico-
        tine in breast milk following the use of cigarettes.)
        Zeitschrift für Kinderheilkunde, 1931, 52, 41-46.

207.   Eneroth, P., Fuxe, K., Gustafsson, J.-Å., Hökfelt, T., Löf-
        ström, A., Skett, P., and Agnati, L. The effect of
        nicotine on central catecholamine neurons and gonado-
        tropin secretion. II. Inhibitory influence of nicotine
        on LH, FSH and prolactin secretion in the ovariectomized
        female rat and its relation to regional changes in dopa-
        mine and noradrenaline levels and turnover. Medical
        Biology, 1977, 55, 158-166.

208.   Eneroth, P., Fuxe, K., Gustafsson, J.-Å., Hökfelt, T., Löf-
        ström, A., Skett, P., and Agnati, L. The effect of
        nicotine on central catecholamine neurons and gonado-
        tropin secretion. III. Studies on prepubertal female
        rats treated with pregnant mare serum gonadotropin.
        Medical Biology, 1977, 55, 167-176.

209.   Erbacher, K., Grumbrecht, P., and Löser, A. Nikotin und
        innere Sekretion. (Nicotine and inner secretion.)
        Archiv für Experimentelle Pathologie und Pharmakologie,
        1940, 195, 121-142.

210.   Ericson, A., Källén, B., and Westerholm, P. Cigarette
        smoking as an etiologic factor in cleft lip and
        palate. American Journal of Obstetrics and Gynecology,
        1979, 135, 348-351.

211.   Eriksson, M., Larsson, G., and Zetterstrom, R. Abuse of
        alcohol, drugs and tobacco during pregnancy--Conse-
        quences for the child. Paediatrician, 1979, 8, 228-242.

212.   Erkkola, R. Physical work capacity of the expectant mother
        and its effect on pregnancy, labor and the newborn.
        International Journal of Gynaecology and Obstetrics,
        1976, 14, 153-159.

213.   Eschwege, E., Papoz, L., Rosselin, G., and Tchobroutsky, C.
        Fetal hypoinsulinism as a cause of small infants of
        smoking mothers? Diabetologia, 1980, 19, 404-405.

214.   Essenberg, J. M. Chronic poisoning of the endocrine glands
        of female albino mice by cigarette smoke. Western
        Journal of Surgery, Obstetrics and Gynecology, 1952,
        60, 635-638.

215.   Essenberg, J. M., Fagan, L., and Malerstein, A. J. Chronic
        poisoning of the ovaries and testes of albino rats and
        mice by nicotine and cigarette smoke. Western Journal
        of Surgery, Obstetrics and Gynecology, 1951, 59,
        27-32.

216.   Essenberg, J. M., Schwind, J., and Patras, A.   The
        effects of nicotine and cigarette smoke on pregnant
        female albino rats and their offsprings.   Journal
        of Laboratory and Clinical Medicine, 1940, 25,
        708-717.

217.   Estel, C. and Kadner, J.   Smoking in pregnancy.
        Zentralblatt für Gynäkologie, 1978, 100, 579-582.

218.   Evans, D. R., Newcombe, R. G., and Campbell, H.   Maternal
        smoking habits and congenital malformations:
        Population study.   British Medical Journal, 1979, 2,
        171-173.

219.   Evans, H. J., Fletcher, J., Torrance, M., and Hargreave,
        T. B.   Sperm abnormalities and cigarette smoking.
        Lancet, 1981, 1, 627-629.

220.   Everson, R. B.   Individuals transplacentally exposed to
        maternal smoking may be at increased cancer risk in
        adult life.   Lancet, 1980, 2, 123-127.

F

221.   Fabia, J. Cigarettes pendant la grossesse, poids de
        naissance et mortalité perinatale. (Effect of cigar-
        ettes on pregnancy, birth weight, and perinatal mortal-
        ity. Canadian Medical Association Journal, 1973, 109,
        1104-1109.

221a.   Fabia, J. and Drolette, M. Twin pairs, smoking in
        pregnancy and perinatal mortality. American
        Journal of Epidemiology, 1980, 112, 404-408.

222.   Fabro, S. and Sieber, S. M. Caffeine and nicotine
        penetrate the pre-implantation blastocyst.
        Nature, 1969, 223, 410-411.

223.   Fardon, H. J. The action of drugs on mammalian uterus.
        Biochemical Journal, 1908, 3, 405-421.

224.   Farrell, J. I. and Lyman, Y. A study of the secretory
        nerves of, and the action of certain drugs on, the
        prostate gland. American Journal of Physiology,
        1937, 118, 64-70.

225.   Fechter, L. D. and Annau, Z. Toxicity of mild prenatal
        carbon monoxide exposure. Science, 1977, 197, 680-
        682.

226.   Fedrick, J. and Adelstein, P. Factors associated with
        low birth weight of infants delivered at term.
        British Journal of Obstetrics and Gynecology, 1978,
        85, 1-7.

227.   Fedrick, J., Alberman, E. D., and Goldstein, H.
        Possible teratogenic effect of cigarette smoking.
        Nature, 1971, 231, 529-530.

228.   Fedrick, J., Alberman, E. D., and Goldstein, H.   Reply
        to Professor Yerushalmy's letter on congenital
        heart disease.   Nature, 1973, 242, 263.

229.   Fedrick, J. and Anderson, A. B. M. Factors associated
        with spontaneous pre-term birth.   British Journal of
        Obstetrics and Gynecology, 1976, 83, 342-350.

230.   Fere, C.   Note sur l'influence de l'exposition prealable
        a la fumée de tabac et aux vapeurs de nicotine sur
        l'incubation de l'oeuf de poule., (Note on the
        influence of early exposure to tobacco smoke and
        nicotine vapor on incubation of the chicken egg.)
        Comptes Rendus des Sciences de la Société de Biologie,
        1893, 45, 948-952.

231.   Fere, C.   De l'influence de la nicotine injectée dans
        l'albumen sur l'incubation de l'oeuf de poule.
        (On the influence of nicotine injected into the
        albumin on incubation of the chicken egg.).
        Comptes Rendus des Sciences de la Société de Biologie,
        1895, 47, 11-13.

232.   Ferguson, B. B., Wilson, D. J., and Schaffner, W.
        Determination of nicotine concentrations in human
        milk.   American Journal of Diseases of Children,
        1976, 130, 837-839.

233.   Fergusson, D. M.   Smoking during pregnancy.   New Zealand
        Medical Journal, 1979, 89, 41-43.

234.   Ferry, J. D., McLean, B. K., and Nikitovitch-Winer, M. B.
        Tobacco-smoke inhalation delays suckling-induced
        prolactin release in the rat.   Proceedings of the
        Society for Experimental Biology and Medicine, 1974,
        147, 110-113.

235.   Fielding, J. E. and Russo, P. K.   Smoking and pregnancy.
        New England Journal of Medicine, 1978, 298, 337-339.

236.   Fielding, J. E., and Yankauer, A.   The pregnancy smoker.
        American Journal of Public Health, 1978, 68, 835-836.

237.   Fischer, H.   Kapillarschaden durch nikotin; eine exper-
        imentelle studie zur frage der pathologie des keim-
        lings und der plazenta.   (Damage to the capillaries
        by nicotine; an experimental study on the pathology
        of the fetus and placenta.)   Zeitschrift für
        Geburtshilfe und Gynäkologie, 1957, 149, 30-65.

238.   Fleig, C.   Influence de la fumée de tabac et de la
        nicotine sur le developpment de l'organisme.
        (Influence of tobacco smoke and nicotine on develop-
        ment of the organism.)   Comptes Rendus de Sciences
        de la Société de Biologie, 1908, 64, 683-685.

239.   Fogelman, K. Smoking in pregnancy and subsequent develop-
        ment of the child. Child: Care, Health and Develop-
        ment, 1980, 6, 233-249.

240.   Forsberg, L., Gustavii, B., Hojerback, T., and Olsson, A. M.
        Impotence, smoking, and beta-blocking drugs. Fertility
        and Sterility, 1979, 31, 589-591.

241.   Forshaw, J. Smoking and pregnancy. British Medical Jour-
        nal, 1972, 2, 406-407.

242.   Franz, K. Studien zur Physiologie des Uterus. (Studies on
        the physiology of the uterus.) Zeitschrift für Geburts-
        hilfe und Gynäkologie, 1904, 53, 361-419.

243.   Frazier, T. M., Davis, G. H., Goldstein, H., and Goldberg,
        I. D. Cigarette smoking and prematurity: A prospective
        study. American Journal of Obstetrics and Gynecology,
        1961, 81, 988-996.

244.   Freour, P. and Coudray, P. Le tabac. Le tabagisme et ses
        consequences. (Tobacco smoking and its consequences.)
        Bordeaux Médicine, 1971, 4, 2509-2582.

245.   Frets, G. P. Keimgifte. (Germ poison.) Archivio e Ras-
        segna Italiana di Ottalmologia, 1930, 24, 91-92.

246.   Friberg, L. Smoking and health. Lancet, 1972, 2, 973.

247.   Fricker, H. S. and Segal, S. Narcotic addiction, pregnancy
        and the newborn. American Journal of Diseases of
        Children, 1978, 132, 360-366.

248.   Fried, P. A. and Oxorn, H. Smoking for Two. Free Press,
        New York, 1980.

249.   Fujita, M. Pharmakologische Untersuchung an den Adnexa
        Uteri in verschiedenen physiologischen Zustanden, mit
        Berücksichtigung des zugehörigen Uterus. (Pharmaco-
        logical investigations on the adnexa of uteri in various
        physiological conditions with reference to the attached
        uterus.) Okayama-Igakkai-Zasshi, 1927, 39, 2025-2050.

250.   Fuxe, K., Agnati, L., Eneroth, P., Gustafsson, J.-Å., Hök-
        felt, T., Löfström, A., Skett, B., and Skett, P. The
        effect of nicotine on central catecholamine neurons and
        gonadotropin secretion. I. Studies in the male rat.
        Medical Biology, 1977, 55, 148-157.

250a.   Fuxe, K., Everitt, B. J., and Hökfelt, T. Enhancement of
        sexual behavior in the female rat by nicotine. Pharma-
        cology, Biochemistry, and Behavior, 1979, 7, 147-151.

G

251.   Garn, S. M., Hoff, K., and McCabe, K. D. Is there
        nutritional mediation of the "smoking effect" on the
        fetus? American Journal of Clinical Nutrition, 1979,
        32, 1181-1184.

252.   Garn, S. M., Johnston, M., Ridella, S. A., and Petzold, A. S.
        Effect of maternal cigarette smoking on Apgar scores.
        American Journal of Diseases of Children, 1981, 135,
        503-506.

253.   Garn, S. M., Petzold, A. S., Ridella, S. A., and Johnston, M.
        Effect of smoking during pregnancy on Apgar and Bayley
        scores in the infant. Lancet, 1980, 2, 912-913.

254.   Garn, S. M., Shaw, H. A., and McCabe, K. D. Relative
        effect of smoking and other variables on size of new-
        born. Lancet, 1977, 2, 667.

255.   Garn, S. M., Shaw, H. A., and McCabe, K. D. Dose response
        effect of maternal smoking. Pediatrics, 1978, 62,
        861-862.

256.   Garn, S. M., Shaw, H. A., and McCabe, K. D. Effect of
        maternal smoking on hemoglobins and hematocrits of
        newborn. American Journal of Clinical Nutrition, 1978,
        31, 557.

257.   Garn, S. M., Shaw, H. A., and McCabe, K. D. Effect of
        maternal smoking on weight and weight gain between
        pregnancies. American Journal of Clinical Nutrition,
        1978, 31, 1302-1303.

258.   Garn, S. M., Shaw, H. A., and McCabe, K. D. Pregnant?
        No ifs, and or butts. Research Staff Physician, 1979,
        25, 152-162.

259.   Garrett, R. J. B. Nicotine and placental iron
         transport. Experientia, 1975, 31, 486-488.

260.   Garvey, D. J. and Longo, L. D. Chronic low level maternal
         carbon monoxide exposure and fetal growth and develop-
         ment. Biology of Reproduction, 1978, 19, 8-14.

261.   Gascon, A. L. and Walaszek, E. J. Mechanism of the
         musculotropic activity of angiotensin on the isolated
         guinea-pig seminal vesicle. Archives International
         de Pharmacodynamie et de Therapie, 1968, 175,
         265-272.

262.   Gatling, R. R. Effect of nicotine on chick embryo.
         Archives of Pathology, 1964, 78, 652-657.

263.   Geller, L. M. Failure of nicotine to affect development
         of offspring when administered to pregnant rats.
         Science, 1959, 129, 212-214.

264.   Genkin, S., Piskarew, D., Serebrjanik, B., and Braun, S.
         Klinik und Pathogenese der Nicotinvergiftung.
         (Clinical pathogenesis of nicotine poisoning.)
         Archives der Klinische Medizin, 1935, 177, 612-660.

265.   Gilani, S. H. Nicotine and cardiogenesis: An experi-
         mental study. Pathologia et Microbiologia, 1971,
         37, 383-392.

266.   Gilani, S. H. Nicotine and cardiogenesis: An histo-
         chemical study. Teratology, 1972, 5, 255-260.

267.   Gilder, S. S. B. Alcohol, tobacco and pregnancy.
         Canadian Medical Association Journal, 1974,
         110, 903-904.

268.   Glass, L., Rajegowda, B. K., Kahn, E. J., and Floyd, M. V.
         Effect of heroin withdrawal on respiratory rate and
         acid-base status in the newborn. New England
         Journal of Medicine, 1972, 286, 746-748.

269.   Godfrey, B. Sperm morphology in smokers. Lancet, 1981,
         1, 948.

270.   Gold, E., Gordis, I., Tonascia, J., and Szkio, M.
         Risk factors for brain tumors in children.
         American Journal of Diseases of Children, 1979,
         109, 309-319.

271.   Goldman, J. A. and Schechter, A. Effect of cigarette
         smoking on glucose tolerance in pregnant women.
         Israel Journal of Medical Science, 1967, 3, 561-
         564.

272.   Goldstein, H. Factors influencing the height of seven-
        year-old children: Results from the national child
        development study. Human Biology, 1971, 43, 92-111.

273.   Goldstein, H. Birthweight and the displacement hypothesis.
        Journal of Epidemiology, 1972, 95, 1-2.

274.   Goldstein, H. Cigarette smoking and low-birthweight
        babies. American Journal of Obstetrics and Gynecology,
        1972, 114, 570-571.

275.   Goldstein, H. Smoking in pregnancy: The statistical con-
        troversy and its resolution. In United States Public
        Health Service. Health Consequences, Education, Ces-
        sation Activities, and Governmental Action. United
        States Department of Health, Education, and Welfare,
        Washington, D. C., 1975. DHEW Publication No. (NIH)
        77-1413.

276.   Goldstein, H. Smoking and pregnancy. Nature, 1973, 245,
        277.

277.   Goldstein, H. Smoking, pregnancy and publicity. Nature,
        1973, 245, 467-468.

278.   Goldstein, H. Smoking in pregnancy: Some notes on the
        statistical controversy. British Journal of Preven-
        tive Medicine, 1977, 31, 13-17.

279.   Goldstein, H., Goldberg, I. D., Frazier, T. M., and
        Davis, G. E. Cigarette smoking and prematurity.
        Public Health Reports, 1964, 79, 553-560.

280.   Gomes, E. P. A slow contracting substance in normal
        human urine. British Journal of Pharmacology, 1955,
        10, 200-207.

280a.   Gordon, B. Sperm morphology in smokers. Lancet, 1981, 1,
        948.

281.   Goujard, J., Kaminski, M., Rumeau-Rouquette, C., and
        Schwartz, D. Maternal smoking, alcohol consumption,
        and abruptio placentae. American Journal of Obstet-
        rics and Gynecology, 1978, 130, 738-739.

282.   Goujard, J., Rumeau-Rouquette, C., and Schwartz, D.
        Smoking during pregnancy, stillbirth, and abruptio
        placentae. Biomedicine, 1975, 23, 20-22.

283.   Graham, H. Smoking in pregnancy: The attitudes of ex-
        pectant mothers. Social Science and Medicine, 1976,
        10, 399-405.

284.   Greiner, I. Nikotinvergiftung, beobachet bei einem
         Saeugling. (Nicotine poisoning observed in a breast
         feeding infant.) Jahrbuch fuer Kinderheilkunde,
         1936, 96, 131-132.

285.   Grumbrecht, P. and Loeser, A. Nikotin und innere
         Sekretion. II. Arbeitsschaden der Frau in Tabak-
         fabriken? (Nicotine and inner secretion. II.
         Work-related damage among women employed in tobacco
         industry?) Archiv fuer experimentelle Pathologie
         und Pharmakologie, 1940, 195, 143-151.

286.   Grumbrecht, P. and Loeser, A. Nicotin und innere Sekretion.
         Erbpathologische Untersuchungen über Keimschadig-
         ungen durch Nicotin. (Nicotine and inner secretion.
         Pathological study of germ poisoning by nicotine.)
         Klinische Wochenschrift, 1941, 2, 853-858.

287.   Guillain, G. and Gy, A. Recherches experimentales sur
         l'influence de l'intoxication tabacique sur la
         gestation. (Experimental studies on the influence
         of tobacco intoxication on pregnancy.) Comptes
         Rendus des Sciences de la Société de Biologie,
         1907, 63, 583-584.

288.   Guiyas, B. G. and Mattison, D. R. Degeneration of mouse
         oocytes in response to polycyclic aromatic hydro-
         carbons. Anatomical Record, 1975, 193, 863-882.

H

289.   Haas, J. F. and Schottenfeld, D. Risks to the offspring
         from parental occupational exposures. Journal of Occu-
         pational Medicine, 1979, 21, 607-613.

290.   Hackett, D. R. Smoking habits during pregnancy. Irish
         Medical Journal, 1979, 72, 483-486.

291.   Haddon, W., Nesbit, R. E. L., and Garcia, R. Smoking and
         pregnancy: Carbon monoxide in blood during gestation
         and at term. Obstetrics and Gynecology, 1961, 18, 262-
         267.

292.   Hagstrom, B. E. and Allen, R. D. The mechanism of nicotine-
         induced polyspermy. Experimental Cell Research, 1956,
         10, 14-23.

293.   Hajeri, H., Spira, A., Frydman, R., and Papiernik-Berkhuer,
         E. Smoking during pregnancy and maternal weight gain.
         Journal of Perinatal Medicine, 1979, 7, 33-38.

294.   Hall, F. Prenatal events and later infant behavior. Jour-
         nal of Psychiatric Research, 1977, 21, 253-257.

295.   Hall, M. H., Pirani, B. B. K., and Campbell, D. The cause
         of the fall in serum folate in normal pregnancy. Brit-
         ish Journal of Obstetrics and Gynaecology, 1976, 83,
         132-136.

296.   Hammer, R. E. and Mitchell, J. A. Effects of nicotine on
         zona pellucida loss and blastocyst development in the
         rat. Anatomical Record, 1979, 194, 629.

297.   Hammer, R. E. and Mitchell, J. A. Nicotine reduces embryo
         growth, delays in implantation, and retards parturition
         in rats. Proceedings of the Society for Experimental
         Biology and Medicine, 1979, 162, 333-336.

298.   Hammer, R. E., Mitchell, J. A., and Goldman, H. Effects of
        nicotine on conceptus development and oviductal/uterine
        blood flow in the rat. Biology of Reproduction (Supple-
        ment 1), 1979, 20, 52A.

299.   Hammond, E. C. Smoking in relation to physical complaints.
        Archives of Environmental Health, 1961, 3, 28-46.

300.   Hamosh, M., Simon, M. R., and Hamosh, P. Effect of nico-
        tine on the development of fetal and suckling rats.
        Biology of the Neonate, 1979, 35, 290-297.

301.   Hannon, S. A Source Book for Conception, Pregnancy, Birth,
        and the First Weeks of Life. Evans Co., New York, 1980.

302.   Hansson, E. and Schmiterlow, C. G. Physiological disposi-
        tion and fate of C^{14}-labelled nicotine in mice and rats.
        Journal of Pharamcology and Experimental Therapeutics,
        1962, 137, 91-102.

303.   Hardy, J. B. and Mellits, E. D. Does maternal smoking
        during pregnancy have a long-term effect on the child?
        Lancet, 1972, 2, 1332-1336.

304.   Hardy, J. B. and Mellits, E. D. Relationship of low birth
        weight to maternal characteristics of age, parity, edu-
        cation and body size. In Reed, D. M. and Stanley, F. J.
        (editors). The Epidemiology of Prematurity. Urban and
        Schwarzenberg, Munich, 1977, 105-118.

305.   Harlap, S. and Davies, A. M. Infant admissions to hospital
        and maternal smoking. Lancet, 1974, 1, 529-532.

306.   Harlap, S. and Davies, A. M. Smoking in pregnancy and
        child development. British Medical Journal, 1974, 2,
        610.

307.   Harlap, S. and Shiono, P. H. Alcohol, smoking and incidence
        of spontaneous abortions in the first and second trimes-
        ter. Lancet, 1980, 2, 173-176.

308.   Harlap, S., Shiono, P. H., Ramcharan, S., Berendes, H., and
        Pellegrin, F. A prospective study of spontaneous fetal
        losses after induced abortions. New England Journal of
        Medicine, 1979, 301, 677-681.

309.   Harries, J. M. and Hughes, T. F. Enumeration of the "crav-
        ings" of some pregnant women. British Medical Journal,
        1958, 2, 39-40.

310.   Harris, R. W., Brinton, L. A., Cowdell, R. H., Skess, D. C.,
        Smith, P. G., Vessey, M. P., and Doll, R. Characteris-
        tics of women with dysplasia or carcinoma in situ of the
        cervix uteri. British Journal of Cancer, 1980, 42, 359-
        369.

311.   Harrison, G. G., Udall, J. N., and Morrow, G. Maternal obes-
        ity, weight gain in pregnancy, and infant birth weight.
        American Journal of Obstetrics and Gynecology, 1980,
        136, 411-412.

312.   Harrison, K. L. The effect of maternal smoking on neonatal
        leucocytes. Australian and New Zealand Journal of Ob-
        stetrics and Gynaecology, 1979, 19, 166-168.

313.   Harrison, K. L. and McKenna, H. Smoking during pregnancy.
        Medical Journal of Australia, 1976, 1, 1020.

314.   Harrison, K. L. and McKenna, H. The effect of maternal
        smoking on cord blood erythrocytes. Australian and New
        Zealand Journal of Obstetrics and Gynecology, 1977, 17,
        160-162.

315.   Hart, S. L. and Mir, M. S. Effects of drugs on human fetal
        intestine: Preliminary investigation. Journal of Phar-
        macy and Pharmacology, 1970, 22, 865-867.

316.   Hasama, B. Recherches pharmacologiques sur le courant elec-
        trique au conduit spermatique isole. (Pharmacological
        studies on electrical current on motility of isolated
        sperm.) Japanese Journal of Medical Science and Pharma-
        cology, 1933, 7, 81-82.

317.   Hatcher, R. A. and Crosby, H. The elimination of nicotine
        in the milk. Journal of Pharmacology and Experimental
        Therapeutics, 1927, 32, 1-6.

318.   Hauser, G. A. Genussmittel in der Schwangerschaft. (Stimu-
        lants during pregnancy.) Therapeutische Umschau, 1971,
        28, 430-434.

319.   Havlicek, V. and Childiaeva, R. Sleep EEG in newborns of
        mothers using alcohol. In Abel, E. L. (editor). Fetal
        Alcohol Syndrome. Volume 2: Human Studies. CRC Press,
        Boca Raton, Florida, 1982, 149-178.

320.   Hawkins, L. H. Blood carbon monoxide levels as a function
        of daily cigarette consumption and physical activity.
        British Journal of Industrial Medicine, 1976, 33, 123-
        125.

321.   Hawkins, L. H., Cole, P. V., and Harris, J. R. Smoking
        habits and blood carbon monoxide levels. Environmental
        Research, 1976, 11, 310-318.

322.   Haworth, J. C. Cigarette smoking during pregnancy and the
        effect upon the fetus. Canadian Journal of Public
        Health, 1973, 64, S20-S24.

323.   Haworth, J. C., Ellestad-Sayed, J. J., King, J., and Dilling,
        L. A. Fetal growth retardation in cigarette-smoking
        mothers is not due to decreased maternal food intake.
        American Journal of Obstetrics and Gynecology, 1980,
        137, 719-723.

324.   Haworth, J. C., Ellestad-Sayed, J. J., King, J., and Dilling,
        L. A. Relation of maternal cigarette smoking, obesity,
        and energy consumption to infant size. American Journal
        of Obstetrics and Gynecology, 1980, 138, 1185-1189.

325.   Haworth, J. C. and Ford, J. D. Comparison of the effects
        of maternal undernutrition and exposure to cigarette
        smoke on the cellular growth of the rat fetus. American
        Journal of Obstetrics and Gynecology, 1972, 112, 653-656.

326.   Hay, D. R. Smoking and health: The 1972 situation.
        New Zealand Medical Journal, 1972, 76, 4-12.

327.   Hayes, F. A., Jenkins, J. H., Feurt, S. D., and Crockford,
        J. A. Observations on the use of nicotine for immobil-
        izing semiwild goats. Journal of the American Veterin-
        ary Association, 1957, 130, 479-482.

328.   Hays, D. P. Teratogenesis: A review of the basic princi-
        ples with a discussion of selected agents. Part II.
        Drug Intelligence and Clinical Pharmacy, 1981, 15, 542-
        566.

329.   Heinonen, O. P., Sloane, D., and Shapiro, S. Birth Defects
        and Drugs in Pregnancy. Publishing Sciences Group,
        Littleton, Massachusetts, 1977.

330.   Hellman, L. M., Johnson, H. L., Tolles, W. E., and Jones,
        E. H. Some factors affecting the fetal heart rate.
        American Journal of Obstetrics and Gynecology, 1961, 82,
        1055-1063.

331.   Hemmenki, K., Mutassen, P., Saloniemi, I., and Luoma, K.
        Congenital malformations and maternal occupation in Fin-
        land: Multivariate analysis. Journal of Epidemiology
        and Community Health, 1981, 35, 5-10.

332.   Hemsworth, B. N. Deformation of the mouse foetus after in-
        gestion of nicotine by the male. IRCS Medical Science
        Library Compendium, 1981, 9, 728-729.

333.   Hemsworth, B. N. Embryopathies due to nicotine referable to
        impairment of spermatogenesis in the mouse. IRCS Med-
        ical Sciences Library Compendium, 1978, 6, 461.

334.   Hemsworth, B. N. and Wardhaugh, A. A. Antifertility action
        of nicotine in the male mouse. IRCS Medical Sciences
        Library Compendium, 1976, 4, 519.

335.   Hemsworth, B. N. and Wardhaugh, A. A. Embryopathies due to nicotine following spermatozoal impairment in Xenopus laevis. IRCS Medical Sciences Library Compendium, 1976, 4, 199.

336.   Hemsworth, B. N. and Wardhaugh, A. A. The mode of action and biological effects of certain antitumor drugs and antifertility agents in Xenopus laevis and Mus musculus. British Journal of Cancer, 1978, 37, 478.

337.   Henderson, B. E., Benton, B., Jung, J., Yu, M., and Pike, M. Risk factors for cancer of the testis in young men. International Journal of Cancer, 1979, 23, 598-602.

338.   Henderson, V. E. and Roepke, M. H. On the mechanism of erection. American Journal of Physiology, 1933, 106, 441-448.

339.   Heron, H. J. The effects of smoking during pregnancy: A review with a preview. New Zealand Medical Journal, 1962, 61, 545-548.

340.   Herriot, A., Billewica, W. Z., and Hytten, F. E. Cigarette smoking in pregnancy. Lancet, 1962, 1, 771-773.

341.   Herscowitz, H. B. and Cooper, R. B. Effect of cigarette smoke exposure on maturation of the antibody response in spleens of newborn mice. Pediatric Research, 1979, 13, 987-991.

342.   Heyer, G. R. Smoking and sexual impotence. Münchener Medizinische Wochenschrift, 1939, 86, 1132.

343.   Hickey, R. J., Boyce, D. E., Clelland, R. C., and Harner, E. B. Smoking and pregnancy. Nature, 1973, 246, 177.

344.   Hickey, R. J., Clelland, R. C., and Bowers, E. J. Maternal smoking, birth weight, infant death, and the self-selection problem. American Journal of Obstetrics and Gynecology, 1978, 131, 805-811.

345.   Hickey, R. J., Clelland, R. C., and Boyce, D. E. Coffee and myocardial infarction. New England Journal of Medicine, 1973, 289, 978.

346.   Hickey, R. J., Clelland, R. C., and Harner, E. B. Smoking, birth-weight, development, and pollution. Lancet, 1973, 1, 270.

347.   Hickey, R. J., Harner, E. B., Clelland, R. C., and Boyce, D. E. Smoking hazards to the fetus. British Medical Journal, 1973, 3, 501.

348.   Hill, E. P., Hill, J. R., Power, G. G., and Longo, L. D.
        Carbon monoxide exchanges between the human fetus and
        mother: Mathematical model. American Journal of
        Physiology, 1977, 232, H311-H323.

349.   Hill, R. M., Craig, J. P., Chaney, M. D., Tennyson, L. M.,
        and McCulley, L. B. Utilization of over-the-counter
        drugs during pregnancy. Clinical Obstetrics and Gynec-
        ology, 1977, 20, 381-394.

350.   Himmelberger, D. U., Brown, B. W., and Cohen, E. N. Cigar-
        ette smoking during pregnancy and the occurrence of
        spontaneous abortion and congenital abnormality. Amer-
        ican Journal of Epidemiology, 1978, 108, 470-479.

351.   Hinds, M. W. and Kolonel, L. M. Maternal smoking and can-
        cer risk to offspring. Lancet, 1980, 2, 703.

352.   Hofstatter, R. Experimentelle Studien über die Einwirkung
        des Nikotins auf die Keimdrusen und auf die Fortpflanz-
        ung. (Experimental studies on the effects of nicotine
        on the gonads and on reproduction.) Virchow's Archives
        für Pathologie und Anatomie, 1923, 244, 183-213.

353.   Hogue, C. J. Coffee in pregnancy. Lancet, 1981, 1, 554.

354.   Hollingsworth, D. R., Moser, R. J., Carlson, J. W., and
        Thompson, K. T. Abnormal adolescent primiparous preg-
        nancy: Association of race, human chorionic somato-
        mammotropin production, and smoking. American Journal
        of Obstetrics and Gynecology, 1976, 126, 230-237.

355.   Hollinshead, W. H. Consequences of smoking in pregnancy.
        Rhode Island Medical Journal, 1979, 62, 207-212.

356.   Holsclaw, D. S. and Topham, A. L. The effects of smoking
        on fetal, neonatal, and childhood development. Pedia-
        tric Annals, 1978, 7, 201-222.

357.   Holste, A. Untersuchungen am überlebenden Uterus. (Examin-
        ation of the enlarged uterus.) Archives für Experimen-
        telle Pathologie und Pharmakologie, 1924, 101, 36-53.

358.   Hook, E. B. A search for the subtle teratogenicity of
        human tobacco smoking. Teratology, 1973, 7, 17A.

359.   Hook, E. B. Consideration of minor birth defects, dermato-
        glyphic abnormalities and asymmetry as possible human
        teratogenic markers. Fourth International Conference
        on Birth Defects, 1974, 91.

360.   Hook, E. B. Changes in tobacco smoking and ingestion of al-
        cohol and caffeinated beverages during early pregnancy:
        Are these consequences, in part, of fetoprotective
        mechanisms diminishing maternal exposure to embryotox-
        ins? In Kelly, S., Hook, E. B., Janerich, D. T., and
        Porter, I. H. (editors). Birth Defects: Risks and
        Consequences, Academic Press, New York, 1976, 173-184.

361.   Hook, E. B., Selvin, S., Garfinkel, J., and Greenberg, M.
        Maternal smoking during gestation and infant morphology
        variation: Preliminary report concerning birth weight
        and incidence of transverse palmar creases. In Janer-
        ich, D. T., Skalko, R. G., and Porter, I. H. (editors).
        Congenital Defects: New Directions in Research, Aca-
        demic Press, New York, 1974, 171-184.

362.   Hopkins, J. Fetal health warning. Food and Cosmetics
        Toxicology, 1979, 17, 172-174.

363.   Hopkins, J. M. and Evans, H. J. Cigarette smoke-induced
        DNA damage and lung cancer risks. Nature, 1980, 283,
        388-390.

364.   Hotovy, R. Versuche zur Frage des Einflusses der chronis-
        chen Nikotinschädigung auf Fruchbarkeit und Nachkommen-
        schaft. (Experiments to determine the effect of chronic
        exposure to nicotine upon fertility and subsequent
        progeny.) Naunyn-Schmiedeberg's Archives of Pathology,
        1948, 205, 54-56.

365.   Howren, H. H. A review of the literature concerning smoking
        during pregnancy. Virginia Medical Monthly, 1965, 92,
        274-279.

366.   Hudson, D. B., Meisami, E., and Timiras, P. S. Brain de-
        velopment in offspring of rats treated with nicotine
        during pregnancy. Experientia, 1973, 29, 286-288.

367.   Hudson, D. B. and Timiras, P. S. Effects of prenatal ad-
        ministration of nicotine on biochemical development of
        the rat brain. Transactions of the American Society of
        Neurochemistry, 1971, 2, 83.

368.   Hudson, D. B. and Timiras, P. S. Nicotine injection during
        gestation: Impairment of reproduction, fetal viability,
        and development. Biology of Reproduction, 1972, 7, 247-
        253.

369.   Hudson, G. S. and Rucker, M. P. Spontaneous abortion. Jour-
        nal of the American Medical Association, 1945, 129, 542.

370.   Hueper, W. C. Experimental studies in cardiovascular path-
        ology. VII. Chronic nicotine poisoning in rats and in
        dogs. American Medical Association Archives of Path-
        ology, 1943, 35, 846-856.

371.   Hunter, J. E. and Haley, D. E. The effect of various con-
        centrations of nicotine in tobacco on the growth and
        development of fowls. Poultry Science, 1930-1931, 10,
        61-67.

372.   Hutton, J. J. and Hackney, C. Metabolism of cigarette
        smoke condensates by human and rat homogenates to form
        mutagens detectable by Salmonella typhimurium TA 1538.
        Cancer Research, 1975, 35, 2461-2468.

373.   Hytten, F. E. Smoking in pregnancy. Developmental Medicine
        and Child Neurology, 1973, 15, 355-357.

374.   Hytten, F. E. Smoking in pregnancy. Reply. Developmental
        Medicine and Child Neurology, 1973, 15, 692.

───────────────J

375. Jacobson, M., Levin, W., and Poppers, P. J.
     Comparison of the O-dealkylation of 7-ethoxycoumarin
     and the hydroxylation of benzo(a)pyrene in human
     placenta. Effect of cigarette smoking. Clinical
     Pharmacology and Therapeutics, 1974, 16, 701-710.

376. Jaffee, O. C. Effects of nicotine on the chick embryo
     heart. International Research Communications
     Systems: Medical Science--Library Compendium,
     1975, 3, 494.

377. James, W. H. Smoking in pregnancy. Nature, 1973,
     246, 235.

378. James, W. H. Smoking in pregnancy and child develop-
     ment. British Medical Journal, 1974, 2, 610-611.

379. Jansson, I. Aetiological factors in prematurity.
     Acta Obstetrica et Gynecologica Scandinavica,
     1966, 45, 279.

380. Jarvinen, P. A. and Osterlund, K. Effect of smoking
     during pregnancy on the fetus, placenta, and
     delivery. Annales Paediatriae Fenniae, 1963,
     9, 18-25.

381. Jedrychowski, W., Malolepszy, A., Piotrowski, J.,
     Chmist-Celinska, B., Glinka, W., and Basta, A.
     Tobacco smoking by pregnant women and birth weight
     of the newborn with reference to the time of
     pregnancy. Polski Tygodnik Lekarski, 1977,
     32, 221-224.

382. Jick, H., Porter, J., and Morrison, A. S. Relation
     between smoking and age of natural menopause.
     Lancet, 1977, 1, 1354-1355.

383.   Johns, W. S. Tobacco, drug and delight. Historical
        Bulletin, 1944, 9, 23-31.

384.   Johnston, C. Cigarette smoking and the outcome of
        human pregnancies: A status report on the con-
        sequences. Clinical Toxicology, 1981, 18, 189-209.

385.   Jones, J. B. The smoking disease. British Medical
        Journal, 1971, 1, 228.

386.   Jones, P. Smoking and pregnancy. Nursing Times,
        1975, 71, 2038-2039.

387.   Joseph, of Cupertino. At The Congregation of Sacred
        Rites on the Beatification and Canonization of
        the Venerable Servant of God, Joseph a Cupertino,
        Professed Priest of the Lesser Conventual Order of
        St Francis (sponsored by) the Most Eminent and
        Reverend Lord Cardinal Casini of Nardo. Responses
        of Fact and of Law to the Objections of the
        Reverend Father, the Advancer of Truth, Concerning
        the Doubt Whether He Possesses the Theological
        Virtues: Faith, Hope, and Charity, and the
        Cardinal Virtues: Prudence, Justice, Fortitude,
        and Temperance, and Instances of his Heroic
        Standing in Each Case. Apostolic Camera, Rome,
        1718.

388.   Juchau, M. R. Human placental hydroxylation of 3,4-
        benzpyrene during early gestation and at term.
        Toxicology and Applied Pharmacology, 1971, 18,
        665-675.

389.   Juchau, M. R., Lee, Q. H., Louviaux, G. L., Symms, K.
        G., Krasner, J., and Yaffe, S. J. Oxidation and
        reduction of foreign compounds in tissues of the
        human placenta and fetus. Fetal Pharmacology,
        1973, 1, 321-334.

K

390.   Kaerki, N. T., Pelkonen,,O., and Tuimala, R. Aryl hydro-
        carbon hydroxylase inducibility in cultured lymph-
        ocytes from smoking and nonsmoking mothers and cord
        blood. Acta Physiologica Scandinavica (Supplement),
        1980, 473, 84.

391.   Kaminski, M., Franc, M., Lebourvier, M., Du Mazaubrun, C.,
        and Rumeau-Rouquette, C. Moderate alcohol use and
        pregnancy outcome. Neurobehavioral Toxicology and
        Teratology, 1981, 3, 173-181.

392.   Kaminski, M., Goujard, J., Rumeau-Rouquette, C. and
        Schwartz, D. Maternal smoking, alcohol consumption,
        and abruptio placentae. American Journal of Obstetrics
        and Gynecology, 1978, 130, 738-739.

393.   Kanaki, S., Hasegawa, K., Mishima, Y., Kobayashi, M.,
        and Motonishi, K. The action of nicotine in the
        egg yolk. Bulletin of the Showa Medical School,
        1957, 17, 21-26. (In Japanese.)

394.   Kanematsu, S. and Sawyer, C. H. Inhibition of the
        progesterone-advanced LH surge at proestrus by
        nicotine. Proceedings of the Society for Experimental
        Biology and Medicine, 1973, 143, 1183-1186.

395.   Kapitulnik, J., Levin, W., and Poppers, P. J. Comparison
        of the hydroxylation of zoxazolamine and benzo(a)-
        pyrene in human placenta: Effect of cigarette smoking.
        Clinical Pharmacology and Therapeutics, 1976, 20,
        557-564.

396.   Karaki, Y. On the influences of nicotine and pyridine
        derivatives on the amount of adrenaline in the adrenal
        glands of the chick embryo. Bulletin of the Showa
        Medical School, 1954, 14, 64-81. (In Japanese.)

397.   Kato, S. Effect of nicotine tartrate and glucuronic acid
        on the vitamin B1 metabolism of chick embryo.
        Folio Pharmacologia Japan 1959, 55, 154-165.

398.   Kato, V., Chihara, K., Ohgo, S., and Imura, H. Effect
        of nicotine on the secretion of growth hormone and
        prolactin in rats. Neuroendocrinology, 1974, 16,
        237-242.

399.   Kaufman, D. W., Slone, D., Rosenberg, L., Miettinen, O. S.,
        and Shapiro, S. Cigarette smoking and age at natural
        menopause. American Journal of Public Health,
        1980, 70, 420-422.

400.   Kehrer, E. Physiologische und pharmakologische Unter-
        suchungen an den überlebenden und lebenden inneren
        Genitalien. (Physiological and pharmacological
        inquiries of longevity and genital function.)
        Archiv fuer Gynaekologie, 1907, 81, 160-210.

401.   Kelly, M. and Roy, F. H. Microcirculatory response of
        fetal mice to maternal nicotine. Clinical Research,
        1971, 19, 322.

402.   Kelsey, J. L., Dwyer, T., Holford, T. R., and Bracken, M. B.
        Maternal smoking and congenital malformations:
        Epidemiological study. Journal of Epidemiology
        and Community Health, 1978, 32, 102-107.

403.   Khan, M. A. Nicotine sulfate-induced skeletal anomalies
        in chick embryos. Teratology, 1975, 11, 25A.

404.   Khan, M. A. Spontaneous vertebral column defects in
        adult chickens and their chemically-induced phenocopies
        in chick embryos. Dissertation Abstracts, 1976,
        36B, 5371-5372.

405.   Khan, M. A., Seibel, W., Gartner, L. P., and Provenza, D. V.
        Effects of nicotine on murine tooth germs in vitro.
        Journal of Dental Research, 1979, 58, 214.

406.   Kier, L. D., Yamasaki, E., and Ames, B. Detection of
        mutagenic activity in cigarette smoke condensates.
        Proceedings of the National Academy of Sciences,
        1974, 71, 4159-4163.

407.   King, J. E. and Becker, R. F. Studies on nicotine ab-
        sorption during pregnancy. I. LD$_{50}$ for pregnant
        and nonpregnant rats. American Journal of Obstetrics
        and Gynecology, 1966, 95, 508-514.

408.   King, J. E. and Dilling, L. A. Fetal growth retardation in
        cigarette-smoking mothers is not due to decreased
        maternal food intake. American Journal of Obstetrics
        and Gynecology, 1980, 137, 719-723.

409.   Kinge, E. The effect of some substances on the isolated
        bull retractor penis muscle. Acta Physiologica
        Scandinavica, 1970, 78, 280-288.

410.   Kirschbaum, T. H., Dilts, P. V., and Brinkman, C. R.
        Some acute effects of smoking in sheep and their
        fetuses. Obstetrics and Gynecology, 1970, 35,
        527-536.

411.   Kitchen, J. M. W. On the health value to man of the
        so-called divinely beneficent gift, tobacco.
        Medical Record, 1889, 35, 459-460.

412.   Kiwaki, T. Influence of nicotine on chick embryo.
        Nippon Yakurigaku Zasshi, 1956, 52, 186-213.
        (In Japanese.)

413.   Kizer, S. Influencia del hábito de fumar sobre el embarazo,
        parto y recién nacido. (Effect of the smoking
        habit on pregnancy, delivery, and the newborn.)
        Revista de Obstetricia y Ginecologia de Venezuela,
        1967, 27, 595-643.

414.   Klein, A. E. and Gorrod, J. W. The metabolism of nicotine
        in cigarette smokers during pregnancy. European
        Journal of Drug Metabolism and Pharmacokinetics,
        1978, 2, 87-93.

415.   Kleinbrecht, J. and Degenhardt, K. H. Causation of
        malformations. Lancet, 1975, 2, 1097-1098.

416.   Kline, J., Stein, Z. A., Susser, M., and Warburton, D.
        Smoking: A risk factor for spontaneous abortion.
        New England Journal of Medicine, 1977, 29, 793-
        796.

417.   Knohira, A. Effects of nornicotine and its related compounds
        on the development of the chick embryo. Showa Igakkai
        Zasshi, 1974, 34, 475-488. (In Japanese.)

418.   Knopf, S. A. Effects of cigarette smoking on tuber-
        culosis among young women, on the child in utero
        and in early life and on certain conditions in
        diseases in adults. Medical Journal and Record,
        1929, 130, 485-489.

419.   Knorr, K. Der Einfluss von Tabak und Alkohol auf Schwanger-
        schaftsverlauf und Kindesentwicklung. (The effect
        of tobacco and alcohol on the course of pregnancy
        and on child development.) Bulletin der Schweizer-
        ischen Akademie der Medizinischen Wissenschaften
        1979, 35, 137-146.

420.   Kolb, P. Exact and detailed description of the Cape of
          Good Hope, containing a very circumstantial account
          of the present state of that celebrated country,
          its settlements, harbor, fortress, form of govern-
          ment, extent, and the regions recently discovered
          in its vicinity. Together with an erudite description
          of the climate and nature of the territory; of its
          animals, fishes, birds, plants, and herbs; likewise
          of various prodigies of Nature discovered in the
          country. To which is added a very accurately compiled
          account of the Hottentots from the author's own
          personal investigations; including a remarkable report
          on their language, religion, manner of living, sin-
          gular traditions, customs, marriage ceremonies,
          circumcisions, and education. Also many other curious
          observations concerning the manners of the nation;
          the condition of the colony of the European inhabitants,
          not to be found in any other description of the
          country. Written with a strict attention to veracity,
          during a long residence in the aforesaid Cape of
          Good Hope, by Peter Kolb, M.A., who was sent to the
          Cape through a distinguished Minister, with letters
          of introduction from the late Right Hon. Lord Nicholas
          Witsen, Burgomaster of the town of Amsterdam, for
          the purposes of this compilation, and for mathematical
          and astronomical research, and who afterward became
          Secretary for Stellenbosch and Drakenstein, and is
          now headmaster of the celebrated school at Neustadt
          on the Asch. Augmented and embellished with useful,
          new, and curious maps, and many illustrations.
          Balthazar Lakeman, Amsterdam, 1927.

421.   Koller, S., Michaelis, H., and Degenhardt, K. H.
          Results of the German study on pregnancy and child
          development. Teratology, 1976, 14, 368.

422.   Kontras, S. B., Salsbury, D., Boden Bender, J. G.,
          Couri, D., Bayer, B., Cordero, L., and Zuspan, F.
          Effect of smoking in pregnant women and their off-
          spring. Pediatric Research, 1976, 10, 331.

423.   Kosdoba, A. S. Zur Frage der experimentellen Pathologie
          der Nebennieren bei intravenoser Nicotineinverleibung.
          (The question of experimental pathology of the
          adrenals by intravenous nicotine.) Archiv fuer
          Klinische Chirurgie, 1929, 156, 550-566.

424.   Kraus, A. S. and Levin, M. L. Cigarette smoking and
          infant survival. American Journal of Obstetrics
          and Gynecology, 1965, 91, 881.

425.   Kretzchmar, R. M. Smoking and health: the role of the
          obstetrician gynecologist. Obstetrics and Gynecology,
          1980, 55, 403-406.

426.   Krieglsteiner, P., Lappy, K., and Fauner, A. Kardio-
        tokographische Untersuchung von Raucherinnen in der
        Schwangerschaft und unter der Geburt. (Cardiological
        study of smokers during pregnancy and their offspring.)
        Medizinische Monatsschrift, 1977, 31, 69-73.

427.   Krishna, K. Tobacco chewing in pregnancy. British
        Journal of Obstetrics and Gynaecology, 1978, 85,
        726-728.

428.   Krous, H. F., Campbell, G. A., Fowler, M. W., Catron, A.
        C., and Farber, J. P. Maternal nicotine administration
        and fetal brain stem damage: A rat model with im-
        plications for sudden infant death syndrome.
        American Journal of Obstetrics and Gynecology,
        1981, 140, 743-746.

429.   Krous, H. F., Fowler, M. W., Catron, A., and Kern, J.
        Maternal nicotine administration and fetal brain stem
        damage: A rat model with implications for sudden
        infant death syndrome. Laboratory Investigation,
        1980, 42, 174.

430.   Kuchle, H. J., Löser, A., Meyer, G., Schmidt, C. G., and
        Sturmer, E. Tabakrauch: Ein Beitrag zur Wirkung von
        Tabakfeuchthaltemitteln. (Tobacco smoke: A contribu-
        tion to the effect of tobacco moisture-holding methods.)
        Zeitschrift für die Gesamte Experimentelle Medizin,
        1952, 118, 554-572.

431.   Kuchle, H. J., Löser, A., Meyer, G., and Sturmer, E. Unter-
        suchungen über Diaethylenglykols als Tabakfeuchthalte-
        mittel. (Studies of diethylene glycol as a means of
        holding moisture in tobacco.) Zeitschrift für die
        Gesamte Experimentelle Medizin, 1952, 119, 266-271.

432.   Kuhnert, P. M., Kuhnert, B. R., and Erhard, P.
        Effect of lead on delta-aminolevulnic acid dehydratase
        activity in maternal and fetal erythrocytes.
        Trace Substances and Environmental Health, 1976,
        10, 373-381.

433.   Kullander, S. and Källén, B. A prospective study of
        smoking and pregnancy. Acta Obstetrica et Gyne-
        cologica Scandinavica, 1971, 50, 83-94.

434.   Kumar, D. and Zourlas, P. A. Studies on human premature
        births. II. In vivo effect of smoking and in vitro
        effect of nicotine on human uterine contractility.
        American Journal of Obstetrics and Gynecology,
        1963, 87, 413-417.

435.   Kuzma, J. W. The Loma Linda study. Paper presented at
        the Fetal Alcohol Syndrome Workshop, Seattle, Washing-
        ton, 1980, May 2-4.

436.   Kuzma, J. W. and Kissinger, D. G. Patterns of alcohol and
        cigarette use in pregnancy. Neurobehavioral Toxicology
        and Teratology, 1981, 3, 211-221.

437.   Kuzma, J. W. and Phillips, R. L. Characteristics of
        drinking and non-drinking mothers. Paper presented
        at the 104th Annual Meeting of the American Public
        Health Association, Miami, Florida, 1976.

438.   Kuzma, J. W. and Phillips, R. L. Characteristics of
        drinking and non-drinking mothers and their offspring.
        Alcoholism: Clinical and Experimental Research, 1977,
        1, 163.

L

439.   Labat, J. B. New journey to the islands of America,
         containing the natural history of these countries,
         the origin, customs, religion, and government of
         the ancient and modern inhabitants; the wars and the
         remarkable events which happened during the long
         stay that the author made there; the commerce and
         the manufactures which have been established there,
         and the methods of increasing them. Work embellished
         by a great number of engraved maps, plans and copper-
         plate illustrations. P. Husson, J. van Duren, T.
         Johsnon, R. Alberts, P. Grosse and C. Le Vier Co.,
         The Hague, 1724.

440.   Lall, K. B., Singhi, S., Gurnani, M., Singhi, P., and
         Garg, O. P. Somatotype, physical growth, and sexual
         maturation in young male smokers. Journal of
         Epidemiology and Community Health, 1980, 34, 295–
         298.

441.   Lambert, B., Lindblad, A., Nordenskjold, M., and
         Werelius, B. Increased frequency of sister chromatid
         exchanges in cigarette smokers. Hereditas, 1978,
         88, 147-149.

442.   Lambert, B., Morad, M., Bridberg, A., Swanbeck, G.,
         and Thyrisson-Hok, M. Sister chromatid exchanges
         in lymphocytes from patients treated with 8-methoxy-
         psoralen and longwave ultraviolet light. Acta
         Dermatovener, 1978, 58, 13-16.

443.   Landauer, W. Nicotine-induced malformations of chicken
         embryos and their bearing on the phenocopy problem.
         Journal of Experimental Zoology, 1960, 143, 107-122.

444.   Landesman-Dwyer, S. and Emanuel, I. Smoking during
         pregnancy. Teratology, 1979, 19, 119-126.

445.   Landesman-Dwyer, S., Keller, L. S., and Streissguth, A. P.
        Naturalistic observations of newborns: Effects of
        maternal alcohol intake. Alcoholism: Clinical and
        Experimental Research, 1978, 2, 171-177.

446.   Landesman-Dwyer, S., Ragozin, A. S., and Little, R. E.
        Behavioral correlates of prenatal alcohol exposure:
        A four-year follow-up study. Neurobehavioral
        Toxicology and Teratology, 1981, 3, 187-193.

447.   Langley, J. N. and Anderson, H. K. On reflex action from
        sympathetic ganglia. Journal of Physiology, 1894,
        16, 410-440.

448.   Langley, J. N. and Anderson, H. K. The innervation of
        the pelvic and adjoining viscera. Journal of
        Physiology, 1895, 19, 71-139.

449.   Larson, P. S., Haag, M. B., and Sylvette, H. Tobacco:
        Experimental and Clinical Studies. Williams and
        Wilkins, Co., Baltimore, 1961.

450.   Larson, P. S. and Silvette, H.(eds.). Tobacco: Experimental
        and Clinical Studies. A Comprehensive Account of
        World Literature. Supplement. Williams and Wilkins,
        Baltimore, 1968.

451.   Larson, P. S. and Silvette, H. (eds.). Tobacco: Experimental
        and Clinical Studies. A Comprehensive Account of
        World Literature. Supplement II. Williams and
        Wilkins, Baltimore, 1971.

452.   Larson, P. S. and Silvette, H. (eds.). Tobacco: Experimental
        and Clinical Studies. A Comprehensive Account of
        World Literature. Supplement III. Williams and
        Wilkins, Baltimore, 1975.

453.   Lasnitzki, I. The effect of a hydrocarbon-enriched
        fraction of cigarette smoke condensate on human fetal
        lung grown in vitro. Cancer Research, 1968, 28,
        510-516.

454.   Laszlo, V. A dohanyzas karos hatasai a gestatios foly-
        amatokra. (The deleterious effects of smoking on
        the sequences of gestation.) Magyar Noorvosok Lapja,
        1969, 32, 163-167.

455.   Lauwerys, R., Buchet, J. P., Roels, H., and Hubermont, G.
        Placental transfer of lead, mercury, cadmium, and
        carbon monoxide in women: I. Comparison of the
        distributions of the biological indices in maternal
        and umbilical cord blood. Environmental Research,
        1978, 15, 278-289.

456.   Lavedan, A. Tratado de Los Usos, Abusos, Propiedades y
        Virtudes del Tabaco, Cafe, te y Chocolate: Extractado
        de Los Mejores Autores Que Han Tratado de Esta Materia,
        a Fin de Que Su Uso No Perjudique a la Salud, Antes
        Bien Pueda Servir de Alivio y Curacion de Muchos Males.
        Por El Lic. Don Antonio Lavedan, Cirujano de Exercito,
        y de la Real Familia de S. M. C. Con Licencia.
        (Treatise on the Uses, Abuses, Qualities, and Virtues
        of Tobacco, Coffee, Tea, and Chocolate. Taken from the
        Best Authors Who Have Dealt with this Subject, So That
        Use of Them May Not Do Harm to Health, But Rather Serve
        as an Alleviation and Cure of Many Ills. By the Licen-
        tiate of Don Antonio Lavedan, Surgeon of the Army and
        of the Royal Family of His Catholic Majesty. With
        Permission.) Royal Printing Shop, Madrid, 1796.

457.   Lazar, P., Gueguen, S., and Boue, J. Epidemiologie des
        avortements spontanées precoces: À propos de 1469
        avortements caryotypes. (Epidemiology of spontaneous
        premature abortions: Study of 1469 karyotyped abor-
        tions.) In Boue, A. and Thibault, C. (eds.). Les
        Accidents Chromosomiques de la Reproduction (Chromo-
        somal Accidents in Reproduction). Institut National
        de la Santé et de la Recherche Médicale, Paris, 1973,
        317-332.

458.   Lee, J. N., Grudzinskas, J. G., and Chard, T. Effect of
        smoking on maternal blood SP$_1$ levels in late preg-
        nancy. Obstetrics and Gynecology, 1981, 57, 220-223.

459.   Lee, Y. C. Experimental studies on the relation between
        nicotine and sexual hormone. Part I. Lethal dose of
        nicotine and sexual difference. Journal of the
        Severance Union Medical College, 1935, 2, 80-86.

460.   Lee, Y. C. Experimental studies on the relatio between
        nicotine and sexual hormone. Part II. Effect of cas-
        tration and sexual hormone on nicotine toxicity.
        Journal of the Severance Union Medical College, 1935,
        2, 87-107.

461.   Lee, Y. C. Experimental studies on the relation between
        nicotine and sexual hormone. Part III. The effects
        of nicotine on the morphological and histological
        changes of female sexual organs after injections of
        female sexual hormone. Journal of the Severance Union
        Medical College, 1935, 2, 108-155.

462.   Lee, Y. C. Experimental studies on the relation between
        nicotine and sexual hormone. Part IV. The antidotal
        action of luteohormone on nicotine toxicity during
        anaphylaxis. Journal of the Severance Union Medical
        College, 1935, 2, 156-159.

463.   Lee, Y. C. The effect of nicotine on sex and sexual hor-
        mone. Chosen Igaku-Kwai Zasshi, 1935, 25, 716-724,
        777-794. (In Japanese.)

464.   Lefkowitz, M. M. Smoking during pregnancy: Long-term
        effects on offspring. Developmental Psychology, 1981,
        17, 192-194.

465.   Lehtovirta, P. and Forss, M. The acute effect of smoking
        on intervillous blood flow of the placenta. British
        Journal of Obstetrics and Gynecology, 1978, 85, 729-
        731.

466.   Lescarbot, M. Nova Francia. (New France.) Translated by
        P. Erondelle. London, 1609.

467.   Leschtschinskaja, O. Toxicology of nicotine. Gigiena
        Truda i Tekh Bezopasnosti, 1926, 7-8, 26-36.
        (In Russian.)

468.   Leschtschinskaja, O. and Tutaev, G. V. Chronic nicotine
        poisoning in experiments with isolated rabbit uteri.
        Gigiena Truda i Tekh Bezopasnosti, 1927, 10, 20-29.
        (In Russian.)

469.   Lewak, N., Van Den Berg, B., and Beckwith, J. B. Sudden
        infant death syndrome risk factors. Clinical Pediatrics,
        1979, 18, 404-411.

470.   Lewin, L. Phantastica: Narcotic and Stimulating Drugs:
        Their Use and Abuse. London, 1931.

471.   Lewis, P. Smoking and pregnancy. Midwife Health Visit
        Community Nurse, 1977, 13, 167, 169-170.

472.   Lickint, F. Der Tabak als Keimgift. (Tobacco as germ
        poison.) Gesundheit und Erziehung, 1934, 47, 35-38.

473.   Lindenschmidt, R. R. and Persaud, T. V. N. Effect of
        ethanol and nicotine in the pregnant rat. Research
        Communications in Chemical Pathology and Pharmacology,
        1980, 27, 195-198.

474.   Lindquist, O. and Bengtsson, C. Menopausal age in relation
        to smoking. Acta Medica Scandinavica, 1979, 205, 73-77.

475.   Lindquist, O. and Bengtsson, C. The effect of smoking on
        menopausal age. Maturitas, 1979, 1, 171-173.

476.   Lindquist, V. A. Carbon monoxide: Its relation to air
        pollution and cigarette smoking. Public Health, 1971,
        86, 20-26.

477.   Little, R. E. Moderate alcohol use during pregnancy and
        decreased infant birth weight. American Journal of
        Public Health, 1977, 67, 1154-1156.

478.   Little, R. E. Maternal alcohol and tobacco use and nausea
        and vomiting during pregnancy: Relation to infant
        birthweight. Acta Obstetrica et Gynecologica Scandin-
        avica, 1980, 59, 495-497.

479.   Little, R. E. Epidemiologic and experimental studies in drinking and pregnancy: The state of the art. Neurobehavioral Toxicology and Teratology, 1981, 3, 163-167.

480.   Little, R. E. and Hook, E. Maternal alcohol and tobacco consumption associated with nausea and vomiting during pregnancy. Acta Obstetrica et Gynecologica Scandinavica, 1979, 15, 15-17.

481.   Livingstone, F. C. Smoking and fetal damage. Science News, 1968, 93, 260.

482.   Löhr, J., Dehnhard, P., and Wehler, V. Zur Morphologie der Plazenta bei Raucherinnen. (Morphology of placentas of female smokers.) Archiv für Gynäkologie, 1975, 219, 376-377.

483.   Long, R. V. and Wolff, W. A. The effect of tobacco on estrus, pregnancy, fetal growth and lactation. North Carolina Medical Journal, 1948, 9, 519-522.

484.   Longo, F. J. and Anderson, E. The effect of nicotine on fertilization in the sea urchin, Arbacia punctulata. Journal of Cellular Biology, 1970, 46, 308-325.

485.   Longo, L. D. Carbon monoxide in the pregnant mother and fetus and its exchange across the placenta. Annals of the New York Academy of Sciences, 1970, 174, 313-341.

485a.   Longo, L. D. Carbon monoxide: Effects on oxygenation of the fetus in utero. Science, 1976, 194, 523-525.

486.   Longo, L. D. Some physiologic effects of carbon monoxide and nicotine on the fetus in utero. In Steinfeld, J., Griffiths, W., Ball, K., and Taylor, R. M. (editors). Public Health Service: Health Consequences, Education, Cessation Activities, and Governmental Action. U. S. Department of Health, Education, and Welfare, Washington, D. C., DHEW Publication No. (NIH) 77-1413, 1977, pp. 211-231.

487.   Longo, L. D. The biological effects of carbon monoxide on the pregnant woman, fetus, and newborn infant. American Journal of Obstetrics and Gynecology, 1977, 129, 69-103.

488.   Longo, L. D. Disorders of placental transfer. In Assali, N. S. and Brinkman, C. R. (editors). Pathophysiology of Gestation. Academic Press, New York, 1972, Volume 2, 1-76.

489.   Lopez, J. A.   Alcohol and tobacco and endocrinal sex
        function.   American Medicine, 1923, 29, 107.

490.   Lowe, C. R.   Effect of mothers' smoking habits on birth
        weight of their children.   British Medical Journal,
        1959, 2, 673-676.

491.   Lubs, M.-L. E.   Racial differences in maternal smoking
        effects on the newborn infant.   American Journal of
        Obstetrics and Gynecology, 1973, 115, 66-76.

492.   Lucas, R. C.   Underdeveloped testes associated with early
        tobacco-chewing.   British Medical Journal, 1882, 2,
        889.

493.   Lux, G. A. and Smith, D. W.   Intrauterine growth deficiency
        syndromes: Proportional reduction in skeletal and
        brain growth.   Clinical Research, 1977, 25, 172A.

M

494.   MacGillivray, I., Rose, G. A., and Rowe, B. Blood pres-
        sure survey in pregnancy. Clinical Science, 1969, 37,
        395-407.

494a.   MacKenzie, K. M. and Angevine, D. M. Infertility in mice
        exposed in utero to benzo(a)pyrene. Biology of Repro-
        duction, 1981, 24, 183-191.

495.   Mackie, A. C. Smoking in pregnancy. British Medical
        Journal, 1974, 2, 55-56.

496.   MacMahon, B., Alpert, M., and'Salber, E. J. Infant weight
        and parental smoking habits. American Journal of
        Epidemiology, 1966, 82, 247-261.

497.   Maddison, R. N. Some effects of smoking in pregnancy.
        Journal of Obstetrics and Gynaecology of the British
        Commonwealth, 1966, 73, 742-746.

498.   Mai, F. M., Munday, R. N., and Rump, E. E. Psychiatric
        interview comparisons between infertile and fertile
        couples. Psychosomatic Medicine, 1972, 34, 431-440.

499.   Malcolm, S. and Shephard, R. J. Personality and sexual
        behavior of the adolescent smoker. American Journal
        of Drug and Alcohol Abuse, 1978, 5, 87-96.

500.   Manning, F. A. and Feyerabend, C. Cigarette smoking and
        fetal breathing movements. British Journal of Ob-
        stetrics and Gynaecology, 1976, 83, 262-270.

500a.   Manning, F. A. and Feyerabend, C. Cigarette smoking and
        fetal breathing movements. Obstetrical and Gyneco-
        logical Survey, 1976, 31, 716-718.

501.   Manning, F. A., Walker, D., and Feyerabend, C. The effect
        of nicotine on fetal breathing movements in conscious
        pregnant ewes. Obstetrics and Gynecology, 1978, 52,
        563-568.

502.   Manning, F. A., Wyn Pugh, E., and Boddy, K.   Effect of
        cigarette smoking on fetal breathing movements in
        normal pregnancies.   British Medical Journal, 1975,
        1, 552-553.

503.   Mantell, C. D.   Smoking in pregnancy: The role played by
        carbonic anhydrase.   New Zealand Medical Journal,
        1964, 63, 601-603.

504.   Marczinski-Verheught, E. and Doerfler, W.   Mutagenic and
        teratogenic effects of cigarette smoking: Summary of
        experimental and clinical observations.   Münchener
        Medizinische Wochenschrift, 1978, 120, 327-330.

505.   Marienfeld, C. J.   Field study relating geochemical en-
        vironment to health and disease.   Annals of the
        New York Academy of Sciences, 1972, 199, 335-348.

506.   Martin, D. C., Barr, H. M., and Streissguth, A. P.   Birth
        weight, birth length, and head circumference related
        to maternal alcohol, nicotine and caffeine use during
        pregnancy.   Teratology, 1980, 21, 54A.

507.   Martin, D. C., Martin, J. C., Streissguth, A. P., and
        Lund, C. A.   Sucking frequency and amplitude in new-
        borns as a function of maternal drinking and smoking.
        In Galanter, M. (ed.).   Currents in Alcoholism.   Vol-
        ume 5:   Biomedical Issues and Clinical Effects of Al-
        coholism.   Grune and Stratton, New York, 1979, 359-366.

508.   Martin, D. C., Streissguth, A. P., and Barr, H. M.   The
        contributions of maternal alcohol, nicotine, and caf-
        feine use to infant birth weight, birth length, and
        head circumference.   Teratology, 1980, 21, 54A.

509.   Martin, J. C.   Maternal alcohol ingestion and cigarette
        smoking and their effects upon newborn conditioning.
        Alcoholism: Clinical and Experimental Research, 1977,
        1, 243-247.

510.   Martin, J. C. and Becker, R. F.   The effects of maternal
        nicotine absorption or hypoxic episodes upon appetitive
        behavior of rat offspring.   Developmental Psychobiology,
        1971, 4, 133-147.

511.   Martin, J. C. and Becker, R. F.   The effects of chronic
        maternal absorption of nicotine or hypoxic episodes
        upon the life span of the offspring.   Psychonomic
        Science, 1972, 29, 145-146.

512.   Martin, J. C., Martin, D. C., and Day-Pfeiffer, H.   The
        interactive effects of maternal nicotine and alcohol
        on rat offspring growth, development and activity.
        Teratology, 1980, 21, 77A.

513.   Martin, J. C., Martin, D. C., Lund, C. A., and Streissguth,
        A. P. Maternal alcohol ingestion and cigarette smok-
        ing and their effects on newborn conditioning. Alco-
        holism: Clinical and Experimental Research, 1977, 1,
        243-247.

514.   Martin, J. C., Martin, D. C., Radow, B., and Day, H. E.
        Growth, development and activity in rat offspring
        following maternal drug exposure. Experimental Aging
        Research, 1976, 2, 235-251.

515.   Martin, J. C., Martin, D. C., Radow, B., and Day, H. E.
        Life span and pathology in offspring following nico-
        tine and methamphetamine exposure. Experimental Aging
        Research, 1979, 5, 509-522.

516.   Martin-Boyce, A., David, G., and Schwartz, D. Alcool,
        tabac et infections genito-urinaires masculines.
        (Alcohol, tobacco, and genitourinary infections in the
        male.) Revue d'Epidemiologie et de Sante Publique,
        1977, 25, 209-216.

517.   Martins, T. and Valle, J. R. Contractilité, survie et
        pharmacologie in vitro de l'epididyme humain. (Con-
        tractility, survival and pharmacology in vitro of the
        human epididymus.) Comptes Rendus des Sciences de la
        Société de Biologie, 1938, 129, 1152-1155.

518.   Martins, T. and Valle, J. R. Pharmacologie comparée des
        canaux deferents et des vescicules seminales, in
        vitro, de rats normaux et de rats castrés. (Com-
        parative pharmacology of the different ducts and
        seminal vesicles of normal and castrated rats, in
        vitro.) Comptes Rendus des Sciences de la Société
        de Biologie, 1938, 127, 1381-1384.

519.   Martins, T., Valle, J. R., and Porto, A. Contractilité
        et reactions pharmacologiques des canaux deferents et
        des vesicules seminales in vitro, de rats castrés et
        traites par les hormones sexuelles. (Contractility
        and pharmacological responses of the different ducts
        and seminal vesicles of castrated rats stimulated by
        sexual hormones in vitro.) Comptes Rendus des
        Sciences de la Société de Biologie, 1938, 127, 1385-
        1388.

520.   Martins, T., Valle, J. R., and Porto, A. Pharmacology in
        vitro of the human vasa deferentia and epididymus:
        The question of the endocrine control of the motility
        of the male accessory genitals. Journal of Urology,
        1940, 44, 682-698.

521.   Matsunaga, E. and Shiota, K. Holoprosencephally in human
        embryos: Epidemiologic studies of 150 cases. Tera-
        tology, 1977, 16, 261-272.

522.   Matsunaga, E. and Shiota, K. Ectopic pregnancy and myoma
        uteri: Teratogenic effects and maternal character-
        istics. Teratology, 1980, 21, 61-69.

523.   Matsunaga, E. and Shiota, K. Search for maternal factors
        associated with malformed human embryos: Prospective
        study. Teratology, 1980, 21, 323-331.

524.   Mattison, D. R. and Thorgiersson, S. S. Smoking and in-
        dustrial pollution, and their effects on menopause
        and ovarian cancer. Lancet, 1978, 1, 187-188.

525.   Mau, G. Nährungs- und Genussmittelkonsum in der Schwanger-
        schaft und seine Auswirkungen auf perinatale Sterb-
        lichkeit, Frühgeburtlichkeit und andere perinatale
        Faktoren. (Subsistence and luxury foods consumption
        during pregnancy and its effect on perinatal mortal-
        ity, prematurity, and other perinatal factors.) Mon-
        atsschrift für Kinderheilkunde, 1974, 122, 539-540.

526.   Mau, G. Rauchen und Schwangerschaft: Die Bedeutung der
        elterlichen Rauchgewohnheiten für das Ungeborene und
        Neugeborene. (Smoking and pregnancy: Importance of
        parental smoking habits for the unborn and the new-
        born.) Medizinische Welt, 1975, 26, 28-30.

527.   Mau, G. Smoking and the fetus. Lancet, 1976, 1 972.

528.   Mau, G. and Netter, P. Die Auswirkungen des väterlichen
        Zigarettenkonsums auf die perinatale Sterblichkeit
        und die Missbildungshäufigkeit. (The effects of
        paternal cigarette smoking on perinatal mortality and
        incidence of malformations.) Deutsche Medizinische
        Wochenschrift, 1974, 99, 1113-1118.

529.   Mau, G. and Netter, P. Kaffee- und Alkoholkonsum--Risiko-
        faktoren in der Schwangerschaft? (Are coffee and al-
        cohol consumption risk factors in pregnancy?) Ge-
        burtshilfe und Frauenheilkunde, 1974, 34, 1018-1022.

530.   Mausner, J. S. Smoking and pregnancy. Annals of Internal
        Medicine, 1973, 79, 272.

531.   Mays, E. E. Cigarette smoking: Its relationship to other
        diseases. Journal of the National Medical Association,
        1973, 65, 520-524.

532.   McCann, J. Smoking mothers damage lifeline to fetus.
        The Journal, 1980, October 1, 4.

533.   McCauley, C. S. Pregnancy After 35. E. P. Dutton,
        New York, 1976.

534.   McConnell, H. Women smokers and health: A long way,
           baby? The Journal, 1978, September 1, 4.

535.   McConnell, H. Smoking major threat to women. The Jour-
           nal, 1980, February 1, 1.

536.   McDonald, R. L. and Lanford, C. F. Effects of
           smoking on selected clinical obstetric factors.
           Obstetrics and Gynecology, 1965, 26, 470-475.

537.   McGarry, J. M. Smoking and leukocyte counts in pregnan-
           cy. British Medical Journal, 1974, 1, 160.

538.   McGarry, J. M. and Andrews, J. Smoking in pregnancy and
           vitamin B_{12} metabolism. British Medical Journal,
           1972, 2, 74-77.

539.   McKean, H. E. Smoking and abortion. New England
           Journal of Medicine, 1978, 298, 113-114.

540.   McKenney, F. D., Essex, H. E. and Mann, F. C. The
           action of certain drugs on the oviduct of the
           domestic fowl. Journal of Pharmacology and
           Experimental Therapeutics, 1932, 45, 113-119.

541.   McLachlan, J. A., Dames, N. M., and Fabro, S.
           Abnormal protein profile in rabbit embryos
           after maternal exposure to some common environmental
           chemicals. Federation Proceedings, 1970, 29,
           348.

542.   McLachlan, J. A., Dames, N. M., Sieber, S. M., and
           Fabro, S. Accumulation of nicotine in the uterine
           fluid of the six-day pregnant rabbit. Fertility
           and Sterility, 1976, 27, 1204-1213.

543.   McLean, B. K., Rubel, A., and Nikitovitch-Winer, M. B.
           The differential effects of exposure to tobacco
           smoke on the secretion of luteinizing hormone
           and prolactin in the proestrous rat. Endocrinology,
           1977, 100, 1561-1570.

544.   McNall, L. K. and Collea, J. V. Environmental
           influences on embryonic and fetal development.
           Current Practice in Obstetrics and Gynecologic
           Nursing, 1978, 2, 67-90.

545.   McRae, B. C. and Choi-Lao, A. National survey on
           smoking and health education in prenatal classes
           in Canada. Canadian Journal of Public Health,
           1978, 69, 427-430.

546.   Meberg, A. What can harm the fetus--tobacco-alcohol-
           drugs? Sykepleien, 1981, 68, 24-30.

547.   Meberg, A., Haga, P., Sande, H., and Foss, O. P.
        Smoking during pregnancy--hematological ob-
        servations in the newborn. Acta Paediatrica
        Scandinavica, 1979, 68, 731-734.

548.   Meberg, A. and Halvorsen, S. Transitory thrombo-
        cytopenia in small-for-dates infants, and in
        newborn mice exposed to hypobaric hypoxia,
        cigarette smoke and CO gas inhalation during
        pregnancy. Paper presented at the Proceedings
        of the European Society for Paediatric Research
        Annual Meeting, Turku, 1978, 58.

549.   Meberg, A., Halvorsen, S., and Örstavik, I.
        Transitory thrombocytopenia in small-for-dates
        infants, possibly related to maternal smoking.
        Lancet, 1977, 2, 303-304.

550.   Meberg, A., Örstavik, I., and Sövde, A. Erythro-
        blastemia and thrombocytopenia in small for
        gestational age infants. Relation to intra-
        uterine hypoxia, infections and maternal smoking.
        Acta Paedriatrica Belgium, 1978, 31, 213.

551.   Meberg, A. and Sande, H. A.   Roking og Graviditet.
        (Smoking and pregnancy.)   Tidsskrift for den
        Norske Laegeforening, 1979, 99, 580-582.

552.   Meberg, A., Sande, H, A., Foss, O. P., and Stenwig, J. T.
        Smoking during pregnancy--Effects on the fetus
        and on thiocyanate levels in mother and baby.
        Acta Paediatrica Scandinavica, 1979, 68, 547-552.

553.   Meiniel, R. Neuromuscular blocking agents and
        axial teratogenesis in the avian embryo.
        Can axial morphogenetic disorders be explained
        by pharmacological action upon muscle tissue.
        Teratology, 1981, 23, 259-271.

554.   Meisami, E. and Hudson, D. B. Effects of chronic
        prenatal administration of nicotine on postnatal
        development of electroconvulsive responses in
        the rat. Federation Proceedings, 1971, 30, 559.

555.   Mellan, J. Smoking and male fertility. Prakticke
        Zubni Lekarstvı, 1967, 47, 890-892.

556.   Mellan, J. Smoking and male sexual defects. Prakticke
        Zubni Lekarstvi, 1963, 43, 862-863.

557.   Melnick, M., Myrianthopoulos, N. C., Bixler, D.,
        and Nance, W. E. Otomandibular anomalies and
        the hemorrhage hypothesis. Teratology, 1977,
        15, 13A.

558.   Menges, R. W., Selby, L. A., Marienfeld, C. J., Aue, A.,
        and Greer, D. L. A tobacco related epidemic of con-
        genital limb deformities in swine. Environmental
        Research, 1970, 3, 285-302.

559.   Meredith, H. V. Relation between tobacco smoking of
        pregnant women and body size of their progeny: A
        compilation and synthesis of published studies.
        Human Biology, 1975, 47, 451-472.

560.   Merritt, T. A. Smoking mothers affect little lives.
        American Journal of Diseases of Children, 1981, 135,
        501-502.

561.   Meyer, M. B. Effects of maternal smoking and altitude on
        birth weight and gestation. In Reed, D. M. and
        Stanley, F. J. (eds.). The Epidemiology of Pre-
        maturity. Urban and Schwarzenberg, Munich, 1977,
        81-104.

562.   Meyer, M. B. How does maternal smoking affect birth
        weight and maternal weight gain? Evidence from the
        Ontario Perinatal Mortality Study. American Journal
        of Obstetrics and Gynecology, 1978, 131, 888-893.

563.   Meyer, M. B. Breast feeding and smoking. Lancet, 1979,
        1, 975-976.

564.   Meyer, M. B. Reply to Rush. American Journal of Obstet-
        rics and Gynecology, 1979, 135, 282-284.

565.   Meyer, M. B. and Comstock, G. W. Maternal cigarette
        smoking and perinatal mortality. American Journal of
        Epidemiology, 1972, 96, 1-10.

566.   Meyer, M. B., Jonas, B. S., and Tonascia, J. A. Perinatal
        events associated with maternal smoking during preg-
        nancy. American Journal of Epidemiology, 1976, 103,
        464-476.

567.   Meyer, M. B. and Tonascia, J. A. Maternal smoking,
        pregnancy complications, and perinatal mortality.
        American Journal of Obstetrics and Gynecology,
        1977, 128, 494-502.

568.   Meyer, M. B., Tonascia, J. A., and Buck, C. The inter-
        relationship of maternal smoking and increased
        perinatal mortality with other risk factors.
        Further analysis of the Ontario perinatal mortality
        study, 1960-1961. American Journal of Epidemiology,
        1974, 100, 443-452.

569.   Mgalobeli, M. Einfluss der Arbeit in der Tabakindustrie
        auf die Geschlechtssphäre der Arbeiterin. (Influence
        of work in tobacco industry on reproduction of female
        workers.) Monatsschrift der Geburtshilfe und
        Gynäkologie, 1931, 88, 237-247.

570.   Miller, H. C. and Hassanein, K. Fetal malnutrition in
        white newborn infants: Maternal factors. Pediatrics,
        1973, 52, 504-511.

571.   Miller, H. C. and Hassanein, K. Maternal factors in
        fetally malnourished black newborn infants. American
        Journal of Obstetrics and Gynecology, 1974, 118, 62-67.

572.   Miller, H. C. and Hassanein, K. Maternal smoking and
        fetal growth of full term infants. Pediatric Re-
        search, 1974, 8, 960-963.

573.   Miller, H. C., Hassanein, K., Chin, T. D Y., and Hens-
        leigh, P. A. Socioeconomic factors in relation to
        fetal growth in white infants. Journal of Pediatrics,
        1976, 89, 638-643.

574.   Miller, H. C., Hassanein, K., and Hensleigh, P. A. Fetal
        growth retardation in relation to maternal smoking
        and weight gain in pregnancy. American Journal of
        Obstetrics and Gynecology, 1976, 125, 55-60.

575.   Miller, H. C., Hassanein, K., and Hensleigh, P. A.
        Effects of behavioral and medical variables on fetal
        growth retardation. American Journal of Obstetrics
        and Gynecology, 1977, 127, 643-648.

576.   Miller, H. C., Hassanein, K., and Hensleigh, P. A.
        Maternal factors in the incidences of low birth weight
        infants among black and white mothers. Pediatric
        Research, 1978, 12, 1016-1019.

577.   Miller, R. K. and Gardner, K. A. Cadmium in the human
        placenta: Relationship to smoking. Teratology, 1981,
        23, 51A.

578.   Miller, R. W. Effect of cigarette smoking on the fetus
        and child. The Committee replies. Pediatrics, 1977,
        60, 766-767.

579.   Mills, C. A. Tobacco smoking: Some hints of its bio-
        logic hazards. Ohio Medical Journal, 1950, 46, 1165-
        1170.

580.   Milne, D. Smoking stunts children's growth--
        before birth. The Journal, 1979, January 1, 5.

581.   Minsker, D. H., Hanson, H. M., Norbury, K. C.,
        and Williams, M. Nicotine infusion into pregnant
        rats affected gestation length, fetal weights and,
        in offspring, behavior, CNS cholinergic and
        anxiolytic binding sites and immunologic com-
        petence. Teratology, 1981, 23, 52A-53A.

582.   Misiewica, L. Cigarette smoking and pregnancy.
        Wiadomosci Lekarskie, 1977, 30, 701-703.

583.   Mitev, P., Peychev, P., Atanasova, D., Atanasova, Z.,
        Peeva, I., and Nikiforov, N. Kum vuprosa za
        vliyanieto na kisloroda i tsigareniya dim
        vurkhu roda i novorodenoto. (Effect of oxygen
        and cigarette smoke on fetus and newborn infant.)
        Akusherstvo i Ginekologiya, 1978, 17, 111-113.

584.   Miyashita, Y. Influence of a theopylline derivative
        on nicotine hydrops in chick embryo. Nippon
        Yakurigaku Zasshi, 1957, 53, 1086-1118. (In
        Japanese.)

585.   Mohr, U. and Althoff, J. Carcinogenic activity of
        aliphatic nitrosamines via the mother's milk
        in the offspring of Syrian golden hamsters.
        Proceedings of the Society for Experimental
        Biology and Medicine, 1971, 136, 1007-1009.

586.   Monson, R. R., Rosenberg, L., Hartz, S.C., Shapiro, S.,
        Heinon, O. P., and Slone, D. Diphenylhydantoin
        and selected congenital malformations.
        New England Journal of Medicine, 1973, 289,
        1049-1052.

587.   Montagu, A. Prenatal Influences. Charles C. Thomas,
        Springfield, Illinois, 1962.

588.   Montilli, P. Sull'andamento della gravidanza
        nell'intossicazione nicotinica. (Influence of
        nicotine on the course of pregnancy.)
        Archivio di Ostetricia e Ginecologia, 1933, 20,
        93-100.

589.   Moore, M. G. Nicotine and the genital glands.
        Münchener Medizinische Wochenschrift, 1936,
        83, 658-659.

590.   Morra, G. Influenza dell'intosscazione nicotinica
        sperimentale sulla gravidanza e sul prodotto del
        concepimento. (Influence of experimental nicotine
        intoxication on pregnancy and the products of
        conception.) Ginecologia, 1935, 1, 996-1022.

591.   Moser, R. J., Hollingsworth, D. R., and Mabry, C. C. Measurement of human chorionic somatomammotropin (HSC) by radioimmunoassay in smokers and nonsmokers. Paper presented at Proceedings of the University of Kentucky Tobacco and Health Research Institute, Tobacco and Health Workshop Conference. Lexington, Kentucky, 1973, March 26-28, 92-108.

592.   Mosier, H. and Armstrong, M. K. Effect of maternal nicotine intake on fetal weight and length in rats. Proceedings of the Society for Experimental Biology and Medicine, 1967, 124, 1135-1137.

593.   Mosier, H. D. and Armstrong, M. K. Effects of maternal intake of nicotine on fetal and newborn rats. Proceedings of the Society for Experimental Biology and Medicine, 1964, 116, 956-958.

594.   Mosier, H. D., Capodanno, C. C., Li, I. O. W., Magruder, C. S., and Jansons, R. A. Resistance of rat fetuses to nicotine-induced lipolysis. Teratology, 1974, 9, 239-245.

595.   Mosier, H. D. and Jansons, R. A. Fate of nicotine in the rat fetus. Teratology, 1972, 5, 263.

596.   Mosier, H. D. and Jansons, R. A. Distribution and fate of nicotine in the rat fetus. Teratology, 1973, 6, 303-311.

597.   Moskovic, S., Tomic, R., Pavlovic, D., Stanojevic, D., and Jonev, M. Uticaj nikotina u trudnice-pusaca na veci procent prevremenih porodjaja. (Effect of nicotine in pregnant smokers on an increase in premature deliveries.) Srpski Arhiv za Celokupno Lekarstvo, 1979, 10, 457-462.

598.   Mukherjee, S. and Mukherjee, S. N. A study of premature births. Indian Journal of Pediatrics, 1971, 38, 389-392.

599.   Mulcahy, R. and Knaggs, J. F. Effect of age, parity and cigarette smoking on outcome of pregnancy. American Journal of Obstetrics and Gynecology, 1968, 101, 844-849.

600.   Mulcahy, R. and Murphy, J. Maternal smoking and the timing of delivery. Journal of the Irish Medical Association, 1972, 65, 175-177.

601.   Mulcahy, R., Murphy, J., and Martin, F. Placental changes and maternal weight in smoking and nonsmoking mothers. American Journal of Obstetrics and Gynecology, 1970, 106, 703-704.

602.   Mullner, J. W. Smoking and health. Canadian Medical
        Association Journal, 1972, 106, 1054.

603.   Murakami, K. The pharmacological studies on the human
        uterus. I and II. Okayama Igakkai Zasshi, 1930, 42,
        2813-2834.

604.   Murdoch, D. E. Birth weight and smoking. Nebraska State
        Medical Journal, 1963, 48, 604-606.

605.   Murotsuka, H. Influence of nicotine on vitamin B_1 metabo-
        lism in the chick embryo. Bulletin of the Showa
        Medical School, 1956, 16, 85-104. (In Japanese.)

606.   Murphy, J. F. and Drumm, J. E. The effects of cigarette
        smoking on the developing fetus. In Greenhalgh, R. M.
        (editor). Smoking and Arterial Disease. Pitman Press,
        Bath, England, 1981, 236-239.

607.   Murphy, J. F., Drumm, J. E., Mulcahy, R. C., and Daly, L.
        The effect of maternal cigarette smoking on fetal
        birthweight and on growth of the fetal biparietal
        diameter. British Journal of Obstetrics and Gynaecol-
        ogy, 1980, 87, 462-466.

608.   Murphy, J. F. and Mulcahy, R. The effect of age, parity,
        and cigarette smoking on baby weight. American Jour-
        nal of Obstetrics and Gynecology, 1971, 111, 22.

609.   Murphy, J. F. and Mulcahy, R. The effects of cigarette
        smoking, maternal age and parity on the outcome of
        pregnancy. Journal of the Irish Medical Association,
        1974, 67, 309-313.

610.   Murphy, J. F. and Mulcahy, R. Cigarette smoking and
        spontaneous abortion. British Medical Journal, 1978,
        1, 988.

611.   Murphy, J. F., Mulcahy, R., and Drumm, J. E. Smoking and
        the fetus. Lancet, 1977, 2, 36.

N

612.   Naeye, R. L.   Effects of maternal cigarette smoking on the fetus and placenta.   British Journal of Obstetrics and Gynaecology, 1978, 85, 732-737.

613.   Naeye, R. L.   Fetal and neonatal disorders related to maternal smoking.   Pediatric Research, 1978, 12, 517.

614.   Naeye, R. L.   Fetal and placental consequences of maternal cigarette smoking.   Laboratory Investigation, 1978, 38, 359.

615.   Naeye, R. L.   Relationship of cigarette smoking to congenital anomalies and perinatal death.   American Journal of Pathology, 1978, 90, 289-293.

616.   Naeye, R. L.   The duration of maternal cigarette smoking, fetal and placental disorders.   Early Human Development, 1979, 3, 229-237.

617.   Naeye, R. L.   Abruptio placentae and placenta previa: Frequency, perinatal mortality, and cigarette smoking.   Obstetrics and Gynecology, 1980, 55, 701-704.

618.   Naeye, R. L.   Cigarette smoking and pregnancy weight gain.   Lancet, 1980, 1, 765-766.

619.   Naeye, R. L.   Influence of maternal cigarette smoking during pregnancy on fetal and childhood growth.   Obstetrics and Gynecology, 1981, 57, 18-21.

620.   Naeye, R. L.   Nutritional/nonnutritional interactions that affect the outcome of pregnancy.   American Journal of Clinical Nutrition, 1981, 34, 727-731.

621.   Naeye, R. L.   Teenaged and pre-teenaged pregnancies: Consequences of the fetal-maternal competition for nutrients.   Pediatrics, 1981, 67, 146-150.

622.   Naeye, R. L., Harkness, W. L., and Utts, J. Abruptio
         placentae and perinatal death: A prospective study.
         American Journal of Obstetrics and Gynecology, 1977,
         128, 740-746.

623.   Naeye, R. L., Ladis, B., and Drage, J. S. Sudden infant
         death syndrome: A prospective study. American
         Journal of Diseases of Children, 1976, 130, 1207.

624.   Naftolin, F. and Usher, R. H. Biological bases and
         consequences of abnormal fetal growth--General intro-
         duction and scope of the problem. In Naftolin, F.
         (editor). Abnormal Fetal Growth: Biological Bases
         and Consequences. Dahlem Konferenzen, Berlin, 1978,
         13-20.

625.   Naguib, S. M., Landin, F. E., and Davis, J. J. Relation
         of various epidemiologic factors to cervical cancer
         as determined by a screening program. Obstetrics
         and Gynecology, 1966, 28, 451-459.

626.   Nagy, L. Lässt sich Nikotin in der Milch rauchender
         Frauen nachweisen? (Can nicotine in the milk of
         smoking women be proved?) Berichte für die Gesamte
         Physiologie und Experimentelle Pathologie, 1934, 81, 562.

627.   Nagy, L. Über den Nikotingehalt der Milch rauchender
         Frauen. (Concerning the nicotine concentration in
         the milk of smoking women.) Pharmazeutische
         Zentralhalle für Deutschland, 1934, 75, 737-740.

628.   Nakazawa, R. Der Einfluss der chronischen Nikotinvergift-
         ung auf die Geschlechtsfunktion der weiglichen Ratten.
         (Influence of chronic nicotine poisoning on sexual
         function of male rats.) Japanese Journal of Medical
         Science, 1931, 5, 109-111.

629.   Nakazawa, R. Der Einfluss der chronischen Nikotin-
         vergiftung auf die Funktion der Geschlechtsorgane
         der weiblichen Ratten. (Influence of chronic nico-
         tine poisoning on the function of the sex organs
         in the female rat.) Japanese Journal of Medical
         Science, 1933, 1, 1-37.

630.   Nanjo, H. Maldevelopment of the fetus caused by nico-
         tine administration during pregnancy and its relation
         to maternal age. Kaibogaku Zasshi, 1964, 39, 212-
         216. (In Japanese.)

631.   Nebert, D. W., Winker, J., and Gelboin, H. V. Aryl
        hydrocarbon hydroxylase activity in human placenta
        from cigarette smoking and nonsmoking women.
        Cancer Research, 1969, 29, 1763-1769.

632.   Neri, A. and Eckerling, B. Influence of smoking and
        adrenaline (epinephrine) on the uterotubal insuflation
        test (Rubin test). Fertility and Sterility, 1969,
        20, 818-828.

633.   Neri, A. and Marcus, S. L. Effect of nicotine on the motil-
        ity of the oviducts in the rhesus monkey: A preliminary
        report. Journal of Reproduction and Fertility, 1972,
        31, 91-97.

634.   Neutel, C. I. and Buck, C. Effect of smoking during
        pregnancy on the risk of cancer in children. Journal
        of the National Cancer Institute, 1971, 47, 59-63.

635.   Neuweiler, W. and Richter, R. H. H. Etiology of gross
        malformations. Schweizerische Medizinische Wochen-
        schrift, 1961, 91, 359-363.

636.   Newcombe, R. G. Cigarette smoking in pregnancy. British
        Medical Journal, 1976, 2, 755.

637.   Newcombe, R. G. and Chalmers, I. Changes in distribution
        of gestational age and birth weight among firstborn
        infants of Cardiff residents. British Medical Jour-
        nal, 1977, 2, 925-926.

638.   Newsweek. Smoking mothers. Newsweek, 1973, 81, 46.

639.   Newsweek. Bad news for women smokers. Newsweek, 1980,
        95, 83.

640.   Nice, L. B. Comparative studies on the effects of
        alcohol, nicotine, tobacco smoke and caffeine on
        white mice. Journal of Experimental Zoology, 1912,
        12, 133-152.

641.   Nichols, P. L. Minimal brain dysfunction: Associated
        with perinatal complications. Paper presented at the
        Society for Research in Child Development, New Orleans,
        Louisiana, 1977.

642.   Nicolov, I. and Chernozemski, I. Tumours in Syrian ham-
        sters following transplacental application of cigarette
        smoke condensate. Paper presented at the XIth Inter-
        national Cancer Congress, Florence, Italy, 1974.

643.   Nicolov, I. and Chernozemski, I.   Tumors and hyperplastic
        lesions in Syrian hamsters following transplacental
        and neonatal treatment with cigarette smoke conden-
        sate. Journal of Cancer Research and Clinical On-
        cology, 1979, 94, 249-256.

644.   Nikonova, T. V.   Transplacental action of benzo(a)pyrene
        and pyrene. Bulletin of Experimental Biology and
        Medicine, 1977, 84, 1025-1027.

645.   Nisbet, I. C. T.   Smoking, pregnancy and publicity.
        Nature, 1973, 245, 468.

646.   Nishimura, H. and Nakai, K.   Developmental anomalies in
        offspring of pregnant mice treated with nicotine.
        Science, 1958, 127, 877-878.

647.   Nishimura, H. and Tanimura, T.   Clinical Aspects of the
        Teratogenicity of Drugs. American Elsevier Publishing
        Company, New York, 1976.

648.   Niswander, K. R. and Gordon, M.   Cigarette smoking.
        In Niswander, K. R. and Gordon, M. (editors). The
        Women and Their Pregnancies: The Collaborative
        Perinatal Study of the National Institute of Neuro-
        logical Diseases and Stroke. W. B. Saunders, Phila-
        delphia, 1972, 72-80.

649.   Niswander, K. R., Singer, J., Westphal, M., and Weiss, N.
        Weight gain during pregnancy and prepregnancy weight.
        Obstetrics and Gynecology, 1969, 33, 482.

650.   Nora, J. J., Nora, A. H., Sommerville, R. J., Hill, R. M.,
        and McNamara, D. G.   Maternal exposure to potential
        teratogens. Journal of the American Medical Associ-
        ation, 1967, 202, 1065-1069.

651.   Norman-Taylor, W. and Dickinson, V. A.   Dangers for
        children in smoking families. Community Medicine,
        1972, 21, 32-33.

652.   Novy, M. J.   Regulation of placental blood flow and
        oxygen transfer in relation to fetal growth.   In
        Naftolin, F. (editor). Abnormal Fetal Growth: Bio-
        logical Bases and Consequences. Dahlem Konferenzen,
        Berlin, 1978, 229-256.

653.   Nylund, L., Lunell, N. O., Persson, B., Fredholm, B. B.,
        and Lagercrantz, H.   Acute metabolic and circulatory
        effects of cigarette smoking in late pregnancy.
        Gynecologic and Obstetric Investigation, 1979, 10,
        39-45.

654.   Nymand, G. Maternal smoking and immunity. Lancet, 1974,
        2, 1379-1380.

655.   Nymand, G. Maternal smoking and neonatal hyperbilirubin-
        aemia. Lancet, 1974, 2, 173.

656.   Obe, G. and Herha, J. Chromosomal aberrations in
         heavy smokers. Human Genetics, 1978, 41, 259-
         263.   .

657.   Obel, E. B. Pregnancy complications following
         legally induced abortion: An analysis of the
         population with special reference to prematurity.
         Danish Medical Bulletin, 1979, 26, 192-199.

658.   Obiang Ossoubita, G. and Loundou Tsoumbou,J. Quatrieme
         Conference Mondiale sur l'Usage du Tabac et
         la Santé, Stockholm 18-21 Juin 1979--Contribution
         à l'Étude du Tabagisme Feminin. (Fourth world
         conference on the use of tobacco and health,
         Stockholm, 18-21.June 1979--Contribution to the
         study of female smoking.)   In Ramstrom, L. M.
         (editor). The Smoking Epidemic, A Matter of
         Worldwide Concern. Almquist and Wiksell Internation-
         al, Stockholm, 1979, 51-53.

659.   Ochsner, A. Influence of smoking on sexuality and
         pregnancy. Medical Aspects of Human Sexuality,
         1971, 5, 81-92.

660.   Ochsner, A. The health menace of tobacco. American
         Scientist, 1971, 59, 246-252.

661.   O'Connell, E. J. and Logan, G. B. Parental smoking
         in childhood asthma. Annals of Allergy, 1974,
         32, 142-145.

662.   Oddoy, A. and Hieronymi, U. Beziehungen zwischen
         sozialen Merkmalen und Verhaltensweisen in der
         Schwangerschaft. 1. Mitteilung: Einfluss
         des Kinderwunsches auf einige Verhaltensweisen
         und Gewohnheiten. (Relationship between social
         characteristics and behavior in pregnancy. 1. The
         effect of planned pregnancy on certain behaviors

and habits.)   Zentralblatt für Gynäkologie, 1978,
100, 877-884.

663.   Oderstedt, I. The Swedish programme: Activities
            at maternity health centers. In Ramstrom, L. M.
            (editor). The Smoking Epidemic, a Matter of
            Worldwide Concern. Almquist and Wiksell
            International, Stockholm, 1979, 278-281.

664.   Oettel, H. Zur Toxikologie des Tabaks und seiner
            Schwelprodukte. (Toxicology of tobaccos and
            their combustion products.) Rehabilitation,
            1972, 25, 7-9.

665.   Ogata, S. Preliminary report of studies on the in-
            fluence of alcohol and nicotine upon the ovary.
            Journal of Medical Research, 1919, 40, 123-127.

666.   Ogier, E. Sulla presenza e sulla reattivita alla
            nicotina di formazioni gangliari nei preparati
            di utero alla Magnus. (Concerning the presence
            and reaction to nicotine on ganglia and the
            uterus.) Archivio Italiano de Scienze Farmacolo-
            giche, 1955, 5, 209-217.

667.   O'Herlihy, C. and Martin, R. H. Screening for
            fetal risk with urinary oestrogen:creatinine
            ratio at 34 weeks. British Journal of Obstetrics
            and Gynaecology, 1980, 87, 388-392.

668.   Ohlendorf, P. Second-hand smoke found guilty.
            The Journal, 1981, April 1, 1.

669.   O'Lane, J. M. Some fetal effects of maternal
            cigarette smoking. Obstetrics and Gynecology,
            1963, 22, 181-184.

670.   Ontario Department of Health. Second Report of
            the Perinatal Mortality Study in Ten University
            Teaching Hospitals. Ontario Department of
            Health. Toronto, 1967.

671.   Ontario Department of Health. Supplement to the
            Second Report of the Perinatal Mortality Study
            in Ten University Teaching Hospitals. Ontario
            Department of Health, Toronto, 1967.

672.   Ott, I. and Scott, J. C. Action of different agents
            upon the secretion of milk. Therapeutic
            Gazette, 1912, 36, 310-313.

673.   Ouchi, H. and Kuroshima, A. Low birth weight
            infants and maternal smoking. Sanfujinka Chiryo
            1970, 21, 1-4. (In Japanese.)

674.   Ouellette, E. M., Rosett, H. L., Rosman, N. P., and
            Weiner, L. Adverse effects on offspring of
            maternal alcohol abuse during pregnancy.
            New England Journal of Medicine, 1977, 297,
            528-530.

675.   Ounsted, M. Maternal constraint of foetal growth
            in man. Developmental Medicine and Child
            Neurology, 1965, 7, 479-491.

P

676.   Paganelli, R., Ramadas, D., Layward, L., Harvey, B. A. M., and Soothill, J. F.   Maternal smoking and cord blood immunity function.   *Clinical and Experimental Immunology*, 1979, 36, 256-259.

677.   Palmer, R., Ouellette, E. M., Warner, L., and Leichtman, S.R.   Congenital malformations in offspring of a chronic alcoholic mother.   *Pediatrics*, 1974, 53, 490-494.

678.   Palmgren, B., Wahlen, T., and Wallander, B.   Toxemia and cigarette smoking during pregnancy: Prospective consecutive investigation of 3,927 pregnancies.   *Acta Obstetrica et Gynecologica Scandinavica*, 1973, 52, 183-185.

679.   Palmgren, B. and Wallander, B.   Cigarettrokning och abort: Konsekutiv prospektiv undersokning av 4312 graviditeter.   (Cigarette smoking and abortion: Consecutive prospective study of 4312 pregnancies.)   *Läkartidningen*, 1971, 68, 2611-2616.

680.   Paulli, S.   *Simonis Paulli, D. Archiatri Regii Danici, & Praelati Aarhusiensis, Medici Consummatissimi, Quadripartitum Botanicum De Simplicium Medicamento Rum Facultatibus Ex Veterum Et Re- Centiorum Decretis Et Observationibus, Cum Medicis, tum Anatomicis, itemque multis Chymica Principia ac Humaniora Studia Spectantibus; In Usus Medicinae Candidatorum Praxim Medicam, Deo Benedicente, Auspicaturorum, Nec non Artis Pharmaceutices Studiosorum concinnatum; Additis 1. Purgantium Dosibus, 2. Guillelmi Laurembergii Botanotheca: jam vero recens auctum 3. Jos. Pitton Turnefort. Charactere Plantarum. 4. Commentario De Usu Et Abusu Tabaci Et Her- Bae Thee: atque multiplicis usus gratia instructum 5. Quintuplici Indice, Latino, Germanico, Danico, Syllabo Authorum Et*

Rerum Locupletissimo, Curante J. Jac. Fickio, PH.
Et M. D. Francofurti ad Maenum, Apud Georgium
Henricum Oehrlingium, Typis, Joh. Baueri, An.
M. DCC. VIII. (Simon Paulli, Royal Danish Court
Physician, Prelate at Aarhus, and consummate
doctor. A Botany in Four Parts Concerning Un-
complicated Medicaments Obtained from Medical and
Anatomical Principles and Observations, and from
Many Chemical Principles and More Learned Studies
of Ancient and Modern Authorities. For the Use
of Candidates in Medicine, About to Begin Medical
Practice, with God's Blessing.Also Prepared for
Those Studying the Art of Pharmacy. With these
Additions. 1. Dosage of Purges; 2. Botanotheca
of William Lauremberg, Now Recently Augmented;
3. Joseph Titton de Tournefort's Characters
of Plants; 4. Commentary Concerning the Use and
Abuse of Tobacco and the Herb Tea; Along with
Instructions for Many Uses; 5. A Five-fold Index
in Latin, German and Danish, a Comprehensive
Syllabus of Authors and Things, Under the
Supervision of J. Jacob Fick, Doctor of Philosophy
and of Medicine.) Georg Heinrich Oehrling Publisher,
Types of John Bauer. Frankfort-on-Main, 1708.

681.   Paun, D.   Der Tabakschaden bein Frauen und Müttern
          und seine Verhütung.   (Tobacco injury in women
          and mothers and its prevention.)   Zeitschrift
          fuer die Gesamte Hygiene und Ihre Grenzgebiete,
          1970, 16, 293-294.

682.   Pavlou, C., Chard, T., Landon, J., and Letchworth,
          A. T.   Circulating levels of human placental
          lactogen in late pregnancy: the effect of
          glucose loading, smoking and exercise.   European
          Journal of Obstetrics, Gynecology, and Reproductive
          Biology, 1973, 3, 45-49.

683.   Pawlowski, A., Olejinik, D., Bem, J., and Roszcynialska,
          M,   Wczesne zmiany histologiczne ukladu nerwowego
          skory krolikow i myszy po pedzlowaniu rozworami
          DMBA, benzenem i acetonem.   (Early histological
          changes of the nervous system of the skin in
          rabbits and mice following application of DMBA
          solutions, benzene and acetone.)   Przeglad
          Dermatologiczny, 1970, 52, 23-29.

684.   Payne, R. W.   Anemia, smoking, and pregnancy.
          British Medical Journal, 1975, 4, 521.

685.   Pechstein, L. A. and Reynolds, W. R. The effect of tobacco
        smoke on the growth and learning behavior of the al-
        bino rat and its progeny. Journal of Comparative
        Psychology, 1937, 24, 459-469.

686.   Peeters, G., Coussens, R., and Sierens, G. Physiology of
        the nerves in the bovine mammary gland. Archives
        Internationales de Pharmacodynamie et de Therapie,
        1949, 79, 75-82.

687.   Pelkonen, O. Environmental influences on human foetal
        and placental xenobiotic metabolism. European Jour-
        nal of Clinical Pharmacology, 1980, 18, 17-24.

688.   Pelkonen, O., Arvela, P., and Karki, N. T. 3,4-benzpyrene
        and N-methylaniline metabolizing enzymes in the immature
        human foetus and placenta. Acta Pharmacologica et
        Toxicologica, 1971, 30, 385-395.

689.   Pelkonen, O., Jouppila, P., and Karki, N. T. Effect of
        maternal cigarette smoking on 3,4-benzpyrene and
        N-methylaniline metabolism in human fetal liver and
        placenta. Toxicology and Applied Pharmacology, 1972,
        23, 399-407.

690.   Pelkonen, O., Jouppila, P., and Karki, N. T. Attempts
        to induce drug metabolism in human fetal liver and
        placenta by the administration of phenobarbital to
        mothers. Archives Internationales de Pharmacodynamie
        et de Therapie, 1973, 202, 288-297.

691.   Pelkonen, O. and Karki, N. T. 3,4-benzpyrene and aniline
        are hydroxylated by human fetal liver but not by
        placenta at 6-7 weeks of fetal age. Biochemical
        Pharmacology, 1973, 22, 1538-1540.

692.   Pelkonen, O., Karki, N. T., Koivisto, M., Tuimala, R., and
        Kauppila, A. Maternal cigarette smoking, placenta
        aryl hydrocarbon hydroxylase and neonatal size. Tox-
        icology Letters, 1979, 3, 331-335.

693.   Pelkonen, O., Karki, N. T., Korhonen, P., Koivisto, M.,
        Tuimala, R., and Kauppila, A. Inducibility of mono-
        oxygenase activities in the human fetus and placenta.
        In Olive, G. (editor). Drug-Action Modification--
        Comparative Pharmacology. Pergamon Press, Oxford,
        1978, 101-111.

694.   Pelkonen, O., Karki, N. T., Korhonen, P., Koivisto, M.,
        Tuimala, R., and Kauppila, A. Human placental aryl
        hydrocarbon hydroxylase: Genetics and environmental
        influences. In Jones, P. W. and Leber, P. (editors).
        Polynuclear Aromatic Hydrocarbons. Ann Arbor Science
        Publishers, Ann Arbor, Michigan, 1979, 765-777.

695.   Penney, D. G., Baylerian, M. S., and Fanning, K. E.
        Temporary and lasting cardiac effects of pre- and
        postnatal exposure to carbon monoxide. Toxicology
        and Applied Pharmacology, 1980, 53, 271-278.

696.   Perazzi, P. Studio sperimentale sui rapporti fra tabagismo
        e gravidanza. (Experimental studies of the effects
        of smoking on pregnancy.) Folia Gynaecologica, 1912,
        7, 295-334.

697.   Perlin, M. J. The epidemiology of drug use during preg-
        nancy. International Journal of the Addictions,
        1979, 14, 355-364.

698.   Perlman, H. H., Dennenberg, A. M., and Sokoloff, N. The
        excretion of nicotine in breast milk and urine from
        cigarette smoking: Its effect on lactation and the
        nursling. Journal of the American Medical Association,
        1942, 120, 1003-1009.

699.   Perraudin, M. L. and Sorin, M. Intoxication probable d'un
        nouveau-né par la nicotine presente dans le lait de sa
        mère. (Probable poisoning of a newborn by nicotine
        present in his mother's milk.) Annales de Pédiatrie,
        1978, 25, 41-44.

700.   Persky, H., O'Brien, C. P., Fine, E., Howard, W. J.,
        Kahn, M. A., and Beck, R. W. The effect of alcohol
        and smoking on testicular function and aggression in
        chronic alcoholics. American Journal of Psychiatry,
        1977, 134, 621-625.

701.   Persson, P. K., Grennert, L., Gennser, G., and Kullander, S.
        A study of smoking and pregnancy with special reference
        to fetal growth. Acta Obstetrica et Gynecologica Scan-
        dinavica, Supplement, 1978, 78, 33-39.

702.   Peters, D. A. V., Taub, H., and Tang, S. Postnatal ef-
        fects of maternal nicotine exposure. Neurobehavioral
        Toxicology, 1979, 1, 221-225.

703.   Peterson, D. R. The sudden infant death syndrome--
        Reassessment of growth retardation in relation to
        maternal smoking and the hypoxia hypothesis. Amer-
        ican Journal of Epidemiology, 1981, 113, 583-589.

704.   Peterson, K. L., Heninger, R. W., and Seegmiller, R. E.
        Fetotoxicity following chronic prenatal treatment of
        mice with tobacco smoke and ethanol. Bulletin of
        Environmental Contamination and Toxicology, 1981, 26,
        813-819.

705.   Peterson, K. L. and Seegmiller, R. E. Fetotoxicity
        following chronic prenatal exposure of mice to ethanol
        and tobacco smoke. Teratology, 1981, 23, 56A.

706.   Peterson, W. F., Morese, K. N., and Kaltreider, D. F.
        Smoking and prematurity: A preliminary report based
        on study of 7,740 Caucasians. Obstetrics and Gynecol-
        ogy, 1965, 26, 775-780.

707.   Petit, G. Les alterations des organes de la génération
        sous l'influence du tabac. (Changes in reproductive
        organs under the influence of tobacco.) Archives
        Générales de Médicine, 1902, 1, 392-394.

708.   Petrakis, N. L., Gruenke, L. D., Beelen, T. C., Castag-
        noli, N., and Craig, J. C. Nicotine in breast fluid
        of nonlactating women. Science, 1978, 199, 303-304.

709.   Pettersson, F. Smoking in pregnancy: Retrospective
        study of the influence of some factors on birth weight.
        Acta Socio-medica Scandinavica, 1969, 1, 13-18.

710.   Pettersson, F. Medicinska skadeverkningar av rokning:
        Rokning och gynekologisk-obstetriska tillstand. (Ad-
        verse clinical effects of smoking: Smoking and gyne-
        cological-obstetrical condition.) Social-Medicinsk
        Tidskrift, 1971, 2, 78-82.

711.   Pettersson, F. Rokning och gynekologisk-obstetriske
        tillstand. (Smoking and gynecological-obstetrical
        condition.) Sykepleien, 1972, 59, 68-70.

712.   Pettersson, F., Fries, H., and Nillius, S. J. Epidemiology
        of secondary amenorrhea. I. Incidence and prevalence
        rates. American Journal of Obstetrics and Gynecology,
        1973, 117, 80-86.

713.   Pettersson, F. and Melander, S. Prediction of birth
        weight: Results of a multiple regression analysis.
        Upsala Journal of Medical Science, 1975, 80, 135-
        140.

714.   Pettersson, F., Melander, S., and Lagerberg, D.
        Perinatal mortality. Acta Paediatrica Scan-
        dinavica, 1973, 62, 221-230.

715.   Pettigrew, A. R., Logan, R. W., and Willocks, J.
        Smoking in pregnancy--Effects on birth weight
        and on cyanide and thiocyanate levels in mother
        and baby. British Journal of Obstetrics and
        Gynecology, 1977, 84, 31-34.

716.   Pfeiffer, C. L. Lobgedichte Auf Den Rauch-Und
        Knaster-Toback. (Facetious panegyric on smoking-
        and canister tobacco.)   Johann Friedrich Schlo-
        mach, Leipzig, 1754.

717.   Pharoah, P. O. D., Alberman, E., Doyle, P., and
        Chamberlain, G. Outcome of pregnancy among
        women in anaesthetic practice. Lancet, 1977,
        1, 34-36.

718.   Phelan, J. P. Diminished fetal reactivity with
        smoking. American Journal of Obstetrics and
        Gynecology, 1980, 136, 230-233.

719.   Phelan, J. P., Elkins, T., and Meguiar, R. V.
        The effects of smoking on the fetal heart rate
        in normal pregnancy. Paper presented at the
        Armed Forces District Meeting of the American
        College of Obstetricians and Gynecologists,
        San Antonio, Texas, September 30-October 5,
        1979.

720.   Philaretes. Work For Chimny-Sweepers. London,
        1601-1602.

721.   Phillips, L. G. Cigarette smoking as a factor in
        sterility. Hawaii Medical Journal, 1943, 2,
        249.

722.   Philone De Conversationibus. Venus Rebutée.
        (Venus Rebutted.)   Cologne, 1722.

723.   Picone, T. A. The Effects of Maternal Weight
        Gain and Cigarette Smoking During Pregnancy
        on Pregnancy Outcome and Neonatal Behavior.
        Ph. D. Dissertation, University of Connecticut,
        1980.

724.   Pirani, B. B. K. Smoking during pregnancy.
        Obstetrical and Gynecological Survey, 1978,
        33, 1-13.

725.   Pirani, B. B. K. and MacGillivray, I. Smoking during
        pregnancy. Its effect on maternal metabolism
        and fetoplacental function. Obstetrics and
        Gynecology, 1978, 52, 257-263.

726.   Pitel, M. and Lerman, S. Further studies on the
        effects of intrauterine vasoconstrictors on
        the fetal rat lens. American Journal of
        Ophthalmology, 1964, 58, 464-470.

727.   Plenefisch, J. D. and Klein, N. W. Teratogenic
        response of cultured rat embryos to serum from
        human cigarette smokers. Teratology, 1980,
        21, 61A-62A.

728.   Pomerance, J. J., Gluck, L., and Lynch, V. A.
        Physical fitness in pregnancy: Its effect on
        pregnancy outcome. American Journal of
        Obstetrics and Gynecology, 1974, 119, 867-876.

729.   Portheine, F. Blutuntersuchungen auf Kohlenmonoxyd
        bei Schwangeren. (Blood tests for carbon
        monoxide in pregnancy women.) Rehabilitation,
        Präventivmedizin, Physikalische Medizin, Sozial-
        medizin, 1972, 25, 24-26.

730.   Powell, J. R. The influence of cigarette smoking
        and sex on theophylline disposition. American
        Review of Respiratory Diseases, 1977, 116, 17-
        23.

731.   Priester, W. A. and Muluihill, J. J. Green-tobacco
        sickness. Lancet, 1975, 1, 803.

732.   Prigge, E. and Hochrainer, D. Effects of carbon
        monoxide inhalation on erythropoiesis and cardiac
        hyperthrophy in fetal rats. Toxicology and
        Applied Pharmacology, 1977, 42, 225-228.

733.   Procianoy, G., Maulaz, P. B., and Schlee, J. C.
        Influencia do fumo durante a gestacao so-re
        o recem-nascido. Resultados e conclusoes da
        observacao humana e da experimentacao animal.
        (Influence of smoking during pregnancy on the
        neonate. Results and conclusions of human
        observations and animal experiments.)
        Pediatria Pratica, 1970, 41, 259-268.

Q

734.   Quick, J. D., Greenlick, M. R., and Roghamnn, K. J.
Prenatal care and pregnancy outcome in an HMO
and general population: a multivariate cohort
analysis. American Journal of Public Health,
1981, 71, 381-390.

735.   Quigley, M. E., Sheehan, K. L., Wilkes, M. M., and
Yen, S. S. C. Effects of maternal smoking on
circulating catecholamine levels and fetal
heart rates. American Journal of Obstetrics
and Gynecology, 1979, 133, 685-690.

R

736.   Rabkin, B. Sin of the mother is visited upon the
        child. Macleans, 1978, 91, 61-62.

737.   Raboch, J. and Mellan, J. Smoking and fertility.
        British Journal of Sexual Medicine, 1975, 2, 35, 37.

738.   Rand, A. Heavy tobacco/pot use continues in pregnancy.
        The Journal, 1981, June 1, 6.

739.   Rantakallio, P. Groups at risk in low birth weight in-
        fants and perinatal mortality: A prospective study
        of the biological characteristics and socioeconomic
        circumstances of mothers in 12,000 deliveries in
        North Finland, 1966. A discriminant function analysis.
        Acta Paediatrica Scandinavica (Supplement 193), 1969,
        1-71.

740.   Rantakallio, P. The assessment of small-for-dates infants
        and associated socio-biological factors. Annales
        Chirurgiae et Gynaecologiae Fenniae, 1973, 62 (Supple-
        ment 184), 1-47.

741.   Rantakallio, P. Relationship of maternal smoking to mor-
        bidity and mortality of the child up to the age of
        five. Acta Paediatrica Scandinavica, 1978, 67, 621-
        631.

742.   Rantakallio, P. The effect of maternal smoking on birth
        weight and the subsequent health of the child.
        Early Human Development, 1978, 2, 371-382.

743.   Rantakallio, P. Social background of mothers who smoke
        during pregnancy and influence of these factors on
        the offspring. Social Science and Medicine, 1979,
        13A, 423-429.

744.   Rantakallio, P., Krause, U., and Krause, K. The use of
        ophthalmological services during the pre-school age,
        ocular findings and family background. Journal of
        Pediatric Ophthalmology and Strabismus, 1979, 15,
        253-258.

745.   Rasmussen, F. Studies in the Mammary Excretion and Ab-
        sorption of Drugs. Carl Fr. Mortenson, Copenhagen,
        1966.

746.   Ravenholt, R. T. and Levinski, M. J. Smoking during
        pregnancy. Lancet, 1965, 1, 961.

747.   Ravenholt, R. T., Levinski, M. J., Nellist, D. J., and
        Takenaga, M. Effects of smoking upon reproduction.
        American Journal of Obstetrics and Gynecology, 1966,
        96, 267-281.

748.   Reckzeh, G., Dontenwill, W., and Leuschner, F. Testing
        of cigarette smoke inhalation for teratogenicity in
        rats. Toxicology, 1975, 4, 289-295.

749.   Redman, C. W. G., Beilin, L. J., Bonnar, J., and Ounsted,
        M. K. Fetal outcome in trial of antihypertensive
        treatment in pregnancy. Lancet, 1976, 2, 753-756.

750.   Reinke, W. A. and Henderson, M. Smoking and prematurity
        in the presence of other variables. Archives of
        Environmental Health, 1966, 12, 600-606.

751.   Reis, K. and Hirsch, H. Bedingungen gesundheitsrelevanter
        Kenntnisse und Verhaltensweisen und ihre Bedeutung
        für die Gesundheitserziehung in der Schwangerschaft.
        (Conditions for relevant health information and
        hygienic behavior and their significance for health
        education in pregnancy.) Zeitschrift für Ärztliche
        Fortbildung, 1980, 74, 330-334.

752.   Rene, A. À propos de l'immunité des bêtes à cornes pour
        la nicotine. Quatre cas d'empoisonnement. (Concerning
        immunity of horned creatures for nicotine. Four cases
        of poisoning.) Gazette des Hôpitaux Civils et Mili-
        taires, 1878, 51, 806.

753.   Resnik, R., Brink, G. W., and Wilkes, M. Catecholamine-
        mediated reduction in uterine blood flow following
        nicotine infusion in the pregnant ewe. Paper pre-
        sented at the Society for Gynecologic Investigation,
        Atlanta, Georgia, March 16-18, 1978.

754.   Resnik, R., Brink, G. W., and Wilkes, M. Catechol-
            amine-mediated reduction in uterine blood flow
            after nicotine infusion in the pregnant ewe.
            Journal of Clinical Investigation, 1979, 63,
            1133-1136.

755.   Reznik, G. and Marquard, G. Effect of cigarette
            smoke inhalation during pregnancy in Sprague-
            Dawley rats. Journal of Environmental Pathology,
            and Toxicology, 1980, 4, 141-152.

756.   Revelli, E. Tabagisme et grossesse. (Tobacco and
            pregnancy.) Minerva Medica, 1961, 52, 708-710.

757.   Rhead, W. J. Smoking and SIDS. Pediatrics, 1977,
            59, 791-792.

758.   Rice, C. and Yoshinaga, K. Effect of nicotine on
            oviducal lactate dehydrogenase during early
            pregnancy in the rat. Biology of Reproduction,
            1980, 23, 445-451.

759.   Rice, J. M. Carcinogenesis: A late effect of ir-
            reversible toxic damage during development.
            Environmental Health Perspectives, 1976, 18,
            133-139.

760.   Richards, I. Retrospective inquiry into possible
            teratogenic effects of drugs in pregnancy.
            Advances in Experimental Medicine and Biology,
            1972, 27, 441-456.

761.   Richmond, A., Bell, M., and Ng, A. Smoking during
            pregnancy. Nursing Mirror, 1975, 141, 50-51.

762.   Riddle, O. and King, C. V. Studies on the physiology
            of reproduction in birds. XII. The relation
            of nerve stimuli to oviducal secretions as
            indicated by effects of atropine and other
            alkaloids. American Journal of Physiology,
            1921, 57, 275-290.

763.   Rio, L. Sulla intossicazione tabagica in gravidanza.
            (Tobacco intoxication in pregnancy.) Annales
            di Ostetricia e Ginecologia, 1925, 47, 266-306.

764.   Ritchie, J. W. K. Fetal breathing and generalized
            fetal movements in normal antenatal patients.
            British Journal of Obstetrics and Gynecology,
            1979, 86, 612-614.

765.   Rivedal, E. and Sanner, T. Synergistic effects of
        smoke extracts, benz(a)pyrene and nickel sulfate
        on morphological transformation of hamster embryo
        cells. Toxicology Letters, 1980, 1000, 17.

766.   Robe, L. B. Just So It's Healthy. CompCare Publishers,
        Minneapolis, Minnesota, 1977.

767.   Robertson, J. S. Birth weight and maternal smoking.
        British Medical Journal, 1959, 2, 1097.

768.   Robinson, J. S. Present methods of intrauterine diag-
        nosis and the need for improvement. In Naftolin, F.
        (editor). Abnormal Fetal Growth: Biological Bases
        and Consequences. Dahlem Konferenzen, Berlin, 1978,
        49-68.

769.   Robinson, P. Yishun nashim burmanyot bizman haheraiom
        vehashpaato alha-em hauber vehaielot. (Smoking
        during pregnancy among Burmese women and its influ-
        ence on mother, fetus, and newborn.) Harefuah,
        1965, 69, 37-39.

770.   Robinson, R. De la pretendue action abortive du tabac.
        (Concerning the alleged abortive action of tobacco.)
        Comptes Rendus des Sciences de la Societe de Bio-
        logie, 1908, 147, 538-539.

771.   Robson, J. M. The problem of teratogenicity. Prac-
        titioner, 1963, 191, 136-142.

772.   Roels, H., Hubermont, G., Buchet, J. P., and Lauwerys, R.
        Placental transfer of lead, mercury, cadmium and
        carbon monoxide in women. 3. Factors influencing
        the accumulation of heavy metals in the placenta
        and the relationship between metal concentration in
        the placenta and in maternal and cord blood. En-
        vironmental Research, 1978, 16, 236-247.

773.   Romaniello, G. Nicotina e prodotto dell concepimento.
        (Ricerche sperimentali dirette e svelare l'even-
        tuale passaggio della nicotina dalla madre al feto.)
        (Nicotine and the products of conception. (Exper-
        imental research directed at revealing the eventual
        passage of nicotine from mother to fetus.) Annales
        di Ostetricia e Ginecologia, 1939, 61, 3-33.

774.   Rosenberg, P. H. and Vanttinen, H. Occupational hazards
        to reproduction and health in anaesthetists and
        paediatricians. Acta Anaesthesiologica Scandinavica,
        1978, 22, 202-207.

775.   Rosenthal, R. N. and Slotkin, T. A. Development of
       nicotinic responses in the rat adrenal medulla
       and long-term effects of neonatal nicotine admin-
       istration. British Journal of Pharmacology, 1977,
       60, 59-64.

776.   Rosett, H. L., Weiner, L., Zuckerman, B., McKinlay, S.,
       and Edelin, K. C. Reduction of alcohol consumption
       during pregnancy with benefits to the newborn.
       Alcoholism: Clinical and Experimental Research,
       1980, 4, 178-184.

777.   Ross, E. M., Butler, N. M., and Goldstein, H. Smoking
       hazards to the fetus. British Medical Journal,
       1973, 4, 51.

778.   Rosso, P. and Luke, B. Influence of maternal weight gain
       on the incidence of fetal growth retardation.
       Clinical Research, 1978, 26, 585A.

779.   Rothschild, L. The fertilization reaction in the sea-
       urchin. The induction of polyspermy by nicotine.
       Journal of Experimental Biology, 1953, 30, 57-67.

780.   Rothschild, L. and Swann, M. M. The fertilization
       reaction in the sea-urchin egg. The effect of nico-
       tine. Journal of Experimental Biology, 1950, 27,
       400-406.

781.   Rowell, P. P. The effect of maternal cigarette smoking
       on the ability of human placental villi to concen-
       trate ɣ-aminoisobutyric acid in vitro. Research
       Communications in Substance Abuse, 1981, 2, 253-266.

782.   Rowell, P. P. and Sastry, B. V. R. Human placental
       cholinergic system: Effects of cholinergic blockade
       on amino acid uptake in isolated placental villi.
       Federation Proceedings, 1977, 36, 981.

783.   Rowell, P. P. and Sastry, B. V. R. The influence of
       cholinergic blockade on the uptake of aminoisobutyric
       acid by isolated human placental villi. Toxicology
       and Applied Pharmacology, 1978, 45, 79-93.

784.   Rowland, T. W., Hubbell, J. P., and Nadas, A. S. Con-
       genital heart disease in infants of diabetic mothers.
       Journal of Pediatrics, 1973, 83, 815-820.

785.   Roy, F. H. and Kelly, M. L. Chronic maternal cigarette
       smoking and infant retrolental fibroplasia: Negative
       results. Annals of Ophthalmology, 1971, 3, 693-694.

786.   Royal College of Physicians. Smoking and Health Now.
        Pitman Medical and Scientific Publishing Company,
        London, 1970.

787.   Ruckebusch, Y. Relationship between the electrical
        activity of the oviduct and uterus of the rabbit
        in vivo. Journal of Reproduction and Fertility,
        1975, 45, 73.

788.   Rudiger, H. W., Kohl, F., Mangels, W., Wichert, V.,
        Bartram, P., Wohler, C. R., and Passarge, E. Benzo-
        pyrene induces sister chromatid exchanges in cul-
        tured human lymphocytes. Nature, 1976, 262, 290-292.

789.   Rumeau-Rouquette, C. Perinatalité et handicaps. (Peri-
        natal period and handicaps.) Revue de Pédiatrie,
        1975, 11, 171-182.

790.   Rumeau-Rouquette, C., Goujard, J., Kaminski, M., Breart, G.,
        Du Mazaubrun, C., Deniel, M., and Hennequin, J. F.
        Mortalité perinatale, antecedents obstétricaux et
        usage du tabac. (Perinatal mortality, obstetrical
        antecedents and use of tobacco.) Journal de Gynéco-
        logie Obstétrique et Biologie de la Reproduction,
        1972, 1, 723-729.

791.   Rumeau-Rouquette, C., Goujard, J., Kaminski, M., Breart, G.,
        Du Mazaubrun, C., Deniel, M., and Hennequin, J. F.
        Risk indicators and environment--Investigations in
        France. In Castelazo-Ayala, L. and MacGregor, C.
        (editors). Gynecology and Obstetrics. Proceedings
        of the World Congress of Gynecology and Obstetrics,
        Mexico City, 1978, 81-95.

792.   Rummler, S. Der Einfluss des Zigarettenrauchens der
        Schwangeren auf Geburtsgewicht und -lange des
        Neugeborene. (Effect of smoking during pregnancy
        on birthweight and length of the newborn.) Zeit-
        schrift für Ärztliche Fortbildung, 1977, 71, 293-
        297.

793.   Rush, D. A correction by the author: Maternal smoking--
        A reassessment of the association with perinatal
        mortality. American Journal of Epidemiology, 1973,
        97, 425.

794.   Rush, D. Examination of the relationship between birth
        weight and cigarette smoking during pregnancy and
        maternal weight gain. Journal of Obstetrics and
        Gynaecology of the British Commonwealth, 1974, 81,
        746-752.

795.   Rush, D. Cigarette smoking during pregnancy: The
        relationship with depressed weight gain and birth
        weight. In Kelly, S., Hook, E. B., Janerich, D. T.,
        and Porter, I. H. (editors). Birth Defects, Risks,
        and Consequences. Academic Press, New York, 1976,
        161-172.

796.   Rush, D. Effects of smoking on pregnancy and newborn
        infants. American Journal of Obstetrics and Gynecol-
        ogy, 1979, 135, 281-282.

797.   Rush, D. Smoking, weight gain, and nutrition during
        pregnancy. American Journal of Obstetrics and
        Gynecology, 1981, 139, 233-234.

798.   Rush, D. and Kass, E. H. Maternal smoking: A reassess-
        ment of the association with perinatal mortality.
        American Journal of Epidemiology, 1972, 96, 183-196.

799.   Rush, D., Stein, Z., and Susser, M. Randomized con-
        trolled trial of prenatal nutritional supplementation
        in New York City. Pediatrics, 1980, 65, 683-697.

800.   Russel, K. P. Eastman's Expectant Motherhood. Little,
        Brown, and Company, Boston, 1977.

801.   Russell, C. S., Taylor, R., and Law, C. E. Smoking in
        pregnancy, maternal blood pressure, pregnancy out-
        come, baby weight and growth and other related
        factors: A prospective study. British Journal of
        Prevention and Social Medicine, 1968, 22, 119-126.

802.   Russell, C. S., Taylor, R., and Maddison, R. N. Some ef-
        fects of smoking in pregnancy. Journal of Obstetrics
        and Gynaecology of the British Commonwealth, 1966,
        73, 742.

803.   Russell, M. A. Cigarette smoking: Natural history of
        a dependence disorder. British Journal of Medical
        Psychology, 1971, 44, 1-16.

804.   Russell, M. A., Wilson, C., and Cole, P. V. Comparison
        of increases in carboxyhaemoglobin after smoking
        "extra-mild" and "non-mild" cigarettes. Lancet,
        1973, 2, 687-690.

805.   Rusu, O., Iorgulescu, M., Deciu, L., and Stambler, S.
        Consideratii asupra adaptarii precoce a nou-nascutului
        dismatur. (Considerations on the early adaptation
        of the immature neonate.) Pediatria, 1973, 22,
        231-243.

806.   Rydin, H. Influence de la nicotine sur l'action
        exercée par l'adrenaline et l'acetyl-choline sur
        l'uterus de lapine. (Influence of nicotine on the
        action exercised by adrenaline and acetyl-choline
        on the uterus of the rabbit.) Comptes Rendus des
        Sciences de la Société de Biologie, 1925, 93, 1193-
        1196.

807.   Rydin, H. Contribution à l'étude pharmacodynamique de
        la nicotine. (Contribution to the pharmacological
        study of nicotine.) Archives Internationales de
        Pharmacodynamie et de Therapie, 1928, 34, 391-441.

S

808.   Said, G. Les effects pathologiques du tabac chez les
       enfants de fumeurs. (Pathological effects of
       tobacco in children of parents who smoke.) Pédiatrie,
       1976, 12, 47-71.

809.   Sánchez Carvajal, M. A. Effects adversos de las drogas
       y otros agentes sobre el feto. (Adverse effects of
       drugs and other agents on the fetus.) Revista de
       Obstetricia y Ginecologia de Venezuella, 1968, 29,
       197-228.

810.   Sapeika, N. The excretion of drugs in human milk--A re-
       review. Journal of Obstetrics and Gynecology of the
       British Commonwealth, 1947, 54, 426-431.

811.   Saracci, R. Smoking during pregnancy. Lancet, 1965,
       1, 1167-1168.

812.   Sastry, B. V. R., Olubadewo, J. O., and Boehm, F. Ef-
       fects of nicotine and cocaine on the release of
       acetylcholine from isolated human placental vilii.
       Archives Internationales Pharmacodynamie et de
       Therapie, 1977, 229, 23-36.

813.   Sato, S., Seino, Y., Ohka, T., Yahagi, T., Nagao, M.,
       Matsushima, T., and Sugimura, T. Mutagenicity of
       smoke condensates from cigarettes, cigars and pipe
       tobacco. Cancer Letters, 1977, 3, 1-8.

814.   Savel, L. E. and Roth, E. Effects of smoking in preg-
       nancy: A continuing retrospective study. Obstetrics
       and Gynecology, 1962, 20, 313-316.

815.   Sawyer, C. Effects of nicotine on pituitary secretion of
       prolactin and luteinizing hormone (LH) in the rat.
       Paper presented at the Third Research Conference
       Committee for Research on Tobacco and Health.
       Newport Beach, California, 1972, May 7-9.

816.   Saxen, I.   Epidemiology of cleft lip and palate:
        An attempt to rule out chance correlations.
        British Journal of Preventative and Social
        Medicine, 1975, 29, 103-110.

817.   Saxton, D. W.   The behaviour of infants whose
        mothers smoke in pregnancy.   Early Human
        Development, 1978, 2, 363-369.

818.   Scanlon, J.   Umbilical cord blood lead concentration.
        Relationship to suburban residency during
        gestation.   American Journal of Diseases of
        Children, 1971, 121, 325-326.

819.   Schafer, E. A. and Mackenzie, K.   The action of
        animal extracts on milk secretion.   Proceedings
        of the Royal Society, Series B, Biological
        Sciences, 1912, 84, 16-22.

820.   Schardein, J. L.   Drugs As Teratogens.   CRC Press,
        Cleveland, Ohio, 1976.

821.   Schievelbein, H.   Biochemischer Wirkungsmechanismus
        des Nikotins oder seiner Abbauprodukte hinischt-
        lich eines eventuellen carcinogenen, mutagenen
        oder teratogenen Effektes.   (Biochemical mechan-
        ism of nicotine or its decomposition products,
        with regard to a possible carcinogenic, muta-
        genic, or teratogenic effect.)   Planta Medica,
        1972, 22, 293-305.

822.   Schildkraut, M. L.   Deadly new facts about women and
        smoking.   Good Housekeeping, 1977, 184, 217-218.

823.   Schimkewitsch, W.   Experimentelle Untersuchungen
        an meroblastischen Eiern.   II. Die Vogel.
        (Experimental investigation of the egg blasto-
        mere.   II. The bird.)   Zeitschrift für
        Wissenschaftliche Zoologie, 1903, 73, 167-277.

823a.   Schinz, H. R. and Slotopolsky, B.   Bemerkungen über
        Entwicklung and Pathologie des Hodens.
        (Observations on the development and pathology
        of the testicle.)   Virchows Archives Abteilung.
        A. Pathologische Anatomie, 1921, 253, 413-420.

824.   Schirren, C.   Die kinderlose Ehe: Möglichkeiten
        und Grenzen der Behandlung aus andrologischer
        Sicht.   (The childless marriage: Possibilities
        and limitations of the treatment from the
        andrological viewpoint.)   Fortschritte der
        Medizin, 1970, 88, 1047-1051.

825.   Schirren, C. Die Wirkung des Nikotins auf die
        Zeugungsfähigkeit des Mannes. (The effect of
        nicotine on the procreative ability of the male.)
        Rehabilitation, Präventivmedizin, Physikalische
        Medizin, Sozialmedizin, 1972, 25, 23-24.

826.   Schirren, C. Importance of follow-up studies in
        andrology. In Hasegawa, T., Hayashi, M., Ebling,
        F. J. G., and Henderson, I. W. (editors). Fertility
        and Sterility. American Elsevier Publishing Com-
        pany, New York, 1973, 210-213.

827.   Schirren, C. Umweltschaden und Fertilität des Mannes:
        Schädigende exogene Einflüsse. (Environmental in-
        fkuences and fertility of the male: Negative
        exogenous influences.) Andrologie, 1973, 5, 91-104.

828.   Schirren, C. Andrologische Aspekte der Sterilität.
        (Andrological aspects of sterility.) Gynäkologische
        Rundschau, 1974, 14 (Supplement 1), 81-90.

829.   Schirren, C. and Gey, G. Der Einfluss des Rauchens auf
        die Fortpflanzungsfähigkeit bei Mann und Frau. (The
        influence of smoking on the reproductive ability of
        men and women.) Zeitschrift für Haut und Geschlechts-
        Krankheiten, 1969, 44, 175-182.

830.   Schlede, E. and Merker, H. J. Effect of benzo(a)pyrene
        treatment on the benzo(a)pyrene hydroxylase activity
        in maternal liver, placenta, and fetus of the rat
        during day 13 to day 18 of gestation. Naunyn-
        Schmiedeberg's Archives of Pharmacology, 1971, 272,
        89-100.

831.   Schlede, E. and Scholz, H. No differences in benzo(a)-
        pyrene hydroxylase activity in the human immature
        placenta and in the human fetal liver from cigarette
        smoking and nonsmoking women. Journal of Perinatal
        Medicine, 1974, 2, 189-195.

832.   Schlipkoter, H. W. and Baginski, B. CEA-Wert bei der
        Bevölkerung in Industriegebieten. (The carcino-
        embryonic antigen in the population of an industrial
        area.) Zentralblatt für Bakteriologie, Parasiten-
        kinde, Infektionskrankheiten und Hygiene, 1976, 16,
        295-303.

833.   Schlumpf, M., Wichtensteiger, W., Maire, R., Shoemaker,
        W. J., and Bloom, F. E. Prenatal development of
        monoamines in the rat and the effect of nicotine.
        Developments in Neuroscience, 1980, 9, 229-230.

834.   Schmidt, F. Aktiv-Rauchen und Passiv-Rauchen also
        schwerwiegende bronchiae Noxe. (Active and passive
        smoking, therefore difficult breathing.) Münchener
        Medizinische Wochenschrift, 1973, 115, 1773-1778.

835.   Schmidt, F. Tabakrauch als wichtigste Luftverschmutzung
        in Innenraumen und als pathogene Noxe fur Passiv-
        raucher. (Tobacco smoking as the most important
        air pollutant for the interior and as a noxious
        pathogen for the passive smoker.) Medizinische
        Welt, 1974, 25, 1824-1832.

836.   Schneider, L. and Henrion, R. Tabac et grossesse.
        (Smoking and body weight.) Journal de Gynécologie,
        Obstétrique, et Biologie de Reproduction, 1979, 8,
        7-12.

837.   Schoeneck, F. J. Cigarette smoking in pregnancy.
        New York State Journal of Medicine, 1948, 41,
        1945-1948.

838.   Schorah, C. J., Zemroch, P. J., Sheppard, S., and
        Smithells, R. W. Leucocyte ascorbic acid and
        pregnancy. British Journal of Nutrition, 1978, 39,
        139-149.

839.   Schramm, W. Smoking and pregnancy outcome. Missouri
        Medicine, 1980, 77, 619-626.

840.   Schroder, B. R. Rauchen in der Schwangerschaft.
        (Smoking during pregnancy.) Deutsche Medizinische
        Wochenschrift, 1933, 59, 1103.

841.   Schwartz, D. Description de l'approche epidemiologique.
        Un example: Le rôle du tabac. (Description of the
        epidemiological approach. An example: The role of
        tobacco.) Archives Françaises de Pédiatrie, 1978,
        35 (Supplement 1), 15-18.

842.   Schwartz, D., Goujard, J., Kaminski, M., and Rumeau-
        Rouquette, C. Smoking and pregnancy: Results of
        a prospective study of 6,989 women. Revue Euro-
        peene d'Études Cliniques et Biologiques, 1972, 17,
        867-879.

843.   Schwarz, R. H. and Yaffe, S. J. (editors). Drugs
        and Chemical Risks to the Fetus and Newborn.
        Alan R. Liss, New York, 1980.

844.   Schwetz, B. A., Smith, F. A., Leong, B. K. J., and
        Staples, R. E. Teratogenic potential of inhaled
        carbon monoxide in mice and rabbits. Teratology,
        1979, 19, 385-392.

845.   Scott, R. B. Some medical aspects of tobacco-smoking.
        British Medical Journal, 1952, 1, 671-675.

846.   Seely, J. E., Zuskin, E., and Bouhuys, A. Cigarette
        smoking: Objective evidence for lung damage in
        teen-agers. Science, 1971, 172, 741-743.

847.   Segal, D. J. Smoking, drinking, and your baby's mental
        health. Mental Retardation Bulletin, 1973, 2,
        64-67.

848.   Sei, K. and Matsumoto, N. Effect of orally administered
        nicotine on intrauterine growth of mice. Teratology,
        1976, 14, 252.

849.   Sei, K. and Matsumoto, N. Effect of orally administered
        nicotine on the intrauterine growth of mice:
        Second report. Teratology, 1978, 18, 147.

850.   Sekiya, Y. On the hydrops of chick embryo induced by
        nicotine. Nippon Yakurigaku Zasshi, 1956, 52, 370-
        397. (In Japanese.)

851.   Seltzer, C. C. Masculinity and smoking. Science, 1959,
        130, 1706-1707.

852.   Senn, S. J. Smoking in pregnancy and low weight babies:
        A statistical consideration. British Journal of
        Prevention and Social Medicine, 1977, 31, 272-273.

853.   Sergueev, G. Au sujet du passage de la nicotine à
        travers le placenta et son influence sur l'état
        de la barrière placentaire. (On the subject of
        nicotine's passage across the placenta and its
        influence on the condition of the placental
        barrier.) Biulletin Exsperimentalnoi Biologii i
        Meditsiny, 1939, 8, 449-453.

854.   Shapiro, S., Siskind, V., Monson, R. R., Heinonen,
        O. P., Kaufman, D. W., and Slone, D. Perinatal
        mortality and birth-weight in relation to aspirin
        taken during pregnancy. Lancet, 1976, 1, 1375-
        1376.

855.   Sheehan, D. and Labate, J. S.   The effect of nico-
            tine on uterine responses to hypogastric nerve
            stimulation.   American Journal of Physiology,
            1942, 137, 456-458.

856.   Shepard, T. H. and Fantel, A. G.   Embryonic and
            early fetal loss.   Clinics in Perinatology,
            1979, 6, 219-243.

857.   Sherif, M. A. F.   The chemical transmitter of the
            sympathetic nerve to the uterus.   Journal
            of Physiology, 1935, 85, 298-308.

858.   Shimoi, S.   Vergleichende Untersuchung über die
            pharmakologische Reaktion des ausgeschnittenen,
            normalen und trachtigen Uterus.   (Comparative
            study of the pharmacologica reaction of the
            excised, normal, and pregnant uterus.)
            Kinki Fujinkwa Gakkai Zassi, 1925, 8, 369.

859.   Shiono, P. H., Harlap, S., Ramcharan, S., Berendes,
            H., Gupta, S., and Pellegrin, F.   Use of
            contraceptives prior to and after conception
            and exposure to other fetal hazards.   Contra-
            ception, 1979, 20, 105-120.

860.   Shiota, K., Chou, M. J., and Nishimura, H.   Factors
            associated with the occurrence of early resorption
            of human embryos.   Mutation Research, 1976,
            38, 347-348.

861.   Shiota, K. and Matsunaga, E.   Epidemiological study
            of holoprosencephaly in human embryos.
            Teratology, 1976, 14, 253.

862.   Shiota, K. and Matsunaga, E.   Genetic and epide-
            miologic study of polydactyly in human embryos
            in Japan.   Jinrui Idengaku Zasshi, 1978, 23,
            173-192.

863.   Shirasuka, Y.   Influence of nicotine and potassium
            iodide on chick embryo.   Bulletin of the Showa
            Medical School, 1957, 17, 56-82.

864.   Sieber, S. M. and Fabro, S.   Identification of
            drugs in the preimplantation blastocyst and
            in the plasma, uterine secretion and urine of the
            pregnant rabbit.   Journal of Pharmacology and
            Experimental Therapeutics, 1971, 178, 65-75.

865.   Silverman, D. T.   Maternal Smoking and Birth
            Weight.   M. A. Thesis.   Johns Hopkins University
            School of Hygiene and Public Health, Baltimore,
            1972.

866.   Silverman, D. T.   Maternal smoking and birth
            weight. American Journal of Epidemiology,
            1977, 105, 513-521.

867.   Silverman, H. M.   Fetal and newborn adverse drug
            reactions.   A survey of the recent literature.
            Intelligence and Clinical Pharmacy, 1974, 8,
            690-693.

868.   Simpson, W. J.   A preliminary report of cigarette
            smoking and the incidence of prematurity.
            American Journal of Obstetrics and Gynecology,
            1957, 73, 808-815.

869.   Sirtori, C., Paganuzzi, M., Lombardo, C., Scalese,
            S., and Ruzzon, T.   Mutagenic substances as
            possible senility factors.   Pharmacological
            Research Communications, 1978, 10, 809-812.

870.   Sisodia, C. S. and Stowe, C. M.   The mechanism of
            drug secretion into bovine milk.   Annals of
            the New York Academy of Sciences, 1964, 11,
            650-661.

871.   Skeveleva, G. and Kiriushchenkov, A.   Effect of
            nicotine on the development of the fetus
            and offspring.   Akush erstvo i Ginekologiya,
            1981, 6, 31-34.   (In Russian.)

872.   Smith, C. S., Rosenfeld, S., and Sacks, L. J.
            Study of the effect of nicotinism in the albino
            rat.   Journal of Pharmacology and Experimental
            Therapeutics, 1935, 55, 274-287.

873.   Smith, D. W.   Growth deficiency disorders--prenatal
            onset.   Major Problems in Clinical Pediatrics,
            1977, 15, 77-84.

874.   Smith, D. W., Harvey, M. A. S., Bunn, B. S., and
            Graham, J. M.   Specific diagnoses and prog-
            noses in SGA infants.   Teratology, 1981, 23,
            62A-63A.

875.   Smith, E. R. and Ilievski, V.   The stimulation of
            canine prostatic secretion by substances with
            ganglion-stimulating actions.   Proceedings
            of the Society for Experimental Biology and
            Medicine, 1969, 130, 667-671.

876.   Smithells, R. W., Ankers, C., Carver, M. E., Lennon,
            D., Schorah, C. J., and Sheppard, S.   Maternal
            nutrition in early pregnancy.   British Journal
            of Nutrition, 1977, 38, 497-506.

877.   Smithells, R. W. and Morgan, D. M.   Transmission
               of drugs by the placenta and the breasts.
               Practitioner, 1970, 204, 14-19.

878.   Snider, A. J. Big smoke, little babies. Science
               Digest, 1969, 65, 52.

879.   Sodano, A.   Ricerche sperimentali sull' influenza
               della nicotina sulla funzione genitale della
               donna.   (Experimental study of the influence
               of nicotine on female sexual function.)
               Archivio di Ostetricia e Ginecologia, 1934,
               21, 559-569.

880.   Sokol, R. J., Miller, S. I., Debanne, S., Golden,
               N., Collins, G., Kaplan, J. and Martier, S.
               The Cleveland NIAAA prospective alcohol-in-
               pregnancy study: The first year. Neurobehavioral
               Toxicology and Teratology, 1981, 3, 203-209.

881.   Sokol, R. J., Miller, S. I., and Reed, G.   Alcohol
               abuse during pregnancy: An epidemiologic study.
               Alcoholism: Clinical and Experimental Research,
               1980, 4, 135-145.

882.   Sontag, L. W. and Wallace, R. F.   The effect of
               cigarette smoking during pregnancy upon the
               fetal heart rate. American Journal of
               Obstetrics and Gynecology, 1935, 29, 77-83.

883.   Soulairac, M. L. and Soulairac, A.   Effect of
               nicotine on the sexual behavior of the male
               rat. Comptes Rendus des Sciences de la Société
               de Biologie, 1972, 166, 798-802.

884.   Soyka, L. F. and Joffe, J. M.   Male mediated drug
               effects on offspring. In Schwarz, R. H. and
               Yaffe, S. J. (editors). Drugs and Chemical
               Risks To The Fetus and Newborn. Alan R. Liss
               Inc., New York, 1980, 49-66.

885.   Spain. Tobacco Monopoly Administration. Consulta
               que Propusieron los Arrendadores del efecto
               del Tabaco, a los firmados en la refolucion
               de ella. (Report of the agents of the tobacco
               monopoly to those signing a resolution about
               it.)   Saragossa, 1698.

886.   Spaur, R. C. and Field, C. A.   Smoking during
               pregnancy. Nebraska Medical Journal, 1980,
               65, 267.

887.   Spellacy, W. N., Buhi, W. C., and Birk, S. A.
        The effect of smoking on serum human placental
        lactogen levels. American Journal of Obstet-
        rics and Gynecology, 1977, 127, 232-234.

888.   Spira, A., Gournier, R., Grob, J. C., Dreyfus, J.,
        and Schwartz, D. Smoking during pregnancy and
        placental blood flow. Paper presented at
        the 6th European Congress of Perinatal Medicine,
        Vienna, 1978.

889.   Spira, A.,and Lazar, P. Spontaneous abortions in
        sibship of children with congenital malform-
        ation or malignant disease. European Journal
        of Obstetrics, Gynecology and Reproductive
        Biology, 1979, 9, 89-95.

890.   Spira, A., Phillippe, E., Spira, N., Dreyfus, J.,
        and Schwartz, D. Smoking during pregnancy and
        placental pathology. Biomedicine, 1977, 27,
        266-270.

891.   Spira, A. and Servent, B. Smoking and the fetus.
        Lancet, 1976, 1, 1416-1417.

892.   Spira, A., Spira, N., Goujard, J., and Schwartz, D.
        Smoking during pregnancy and placental weight.
        A multivariate analysis on 3759 cases. Journal
        of Perinatal Medicine, 1975, 3, 237-241.

893.   Sram, R. J. Geneticke riziko koureni. (Genetic
        risk of smoking.)   Prakticky Lekar, 1981,
        61, 49-53.

894.   Stadtlander, K. H. Über die Wirkung des Nicotins
        auf Reimdrusen und Nebennieren.(Concerning
        the effects of nicotine on glands and adrenals.)
        Zeitschrift fuer die Gesamte Experimentelle
        Medizin, 1936, 99, 670-680.

895.   Stalhandske, T., Slanina, P., Tjalve, H., Hansson,
        E., and Schmiterlow, C. G. Metabolism in vitro
        of ^{14}C-nicotine in livers of foetal, newborn,
        and young mice. Acta Pharmacologica et Tox-
        icologica, 1969, 27, 363-380.

896.   Stark, R. The Book of Aphrodisiacs. Stein and Day,
        New York, 1980.

897.   Steele, R., Kraus, A.S., and Langworth, J. T.
        Sudden, unexpected death in infancy in Ontario.
        Part I. Methodology and findings related to
        the host. Canadian Journal of Public Health,
        1967, 58, 359-371.

898.   Steele, T. and Langworth, J. T.   The relationship
           of antenatal and postnatal factors to sudden
           unexpected death in infancy.   Canadian Medical
           Association Journal, 1966, 94, 1165-1171.

899.   Stekhun, F. I.   'Alkogol' i tabkourniye kak voz-
           mozhnyye prichiny besplodiya muzhchin.
           ('Alcohol' and tobacco smoking as possible
           causes of sterility in males.).   Vestnik
           Dermatologii i Venerologii, 1979, 7, 61-65.

900.   Stella, B.   Il Tobacco.   Opera Di D. Benedetto
           Stella Da Civita Cāstellana M.D.S.B.   Nella
           Quale Si Tratta Dell'Origine, Historia,
           Coltura, Preparatione, Qualita, Natura, Virtu,
           & Uso In Fumo, In Poluere, In Foglia, In
           Lambitiuo, Et In Medicina.   Della Pianta
           Volgarmente Detta Tabacco.   Si Discorre Degl'
           Utili Ch'arreca Moderatamente Preso, De I
           Danni Ch'apporta Moderatamente Usato, E Qual
           Fia Il Vero, E Legitimo Trattato Naturale,
           Medico, Morae, E Curioso.   (Tobacco.   Works of
           Benedetto Stella, of Civita Castellan, M.D.S.B.
           In which are Treated the Origin, History, Cul-
           ture, Preparation, Quality, Nature, Virtue,
           and Use in Smoke, Snuff, Leaf, Lambative, and
           in Medicine.   Discussing its utility When
           Used in Moderation, Its Harmfulness When Used
           Immoderately, and of the True and Proper Way
           of Taking It.   A Natural, Medical, Moral, and
           Curious Treatise.)   Filippo Maria Mancini,
           Rome, 1669.

901.   Sterling, T. D. and Kobayashi, D.   A critical
           review of reports on the effects of smoking
           on sex and fertility.   Journal of Sex Research,
           1975, 11, 201-217.

902.   Stevenson, R. E.   The Fetus and Newly Born Infant:
           Influences of the Prenatal Environment.
           C. V. Mosby, St. Louis, 1973.

903.   Stewart, A., Webb, J., and Hewitt, D.   A survey
           of childhood malignancies.   British Medical
           Journal, 1958, 1, 1495-1508.

904.   Streissguth, A. P., Barr, H. M., Martin, D. C.,
           and Herman, C.   Effects of maternal alcohol,
           nicotine, and caffeine use during pregnancy
           on infant development at eight months.   Al-
           coholism: Clinical and Experimental Research,
           1979, 3, 197.

905.   Streissguth, A. P., Barr, H. M., Martin, D. C., and
        Herman, C. S. Effects of maternal alcohol, nico-
        tine and caffeine use during pregnancy on in-
        fant development at eight months. Paper
        presented at the biennial meeting of the
        Society for Research in Child Development,
        San Francisoo, 1979.

906.   Streissguth, A. P., Barr, H. M., Martin, D. C.,
        and Herman, C. S. Effects of maternal alcohol,
        nicotine and caffeine use during pregnancy on
        infant mental and motor development at 8
        months. Alcoholism: Clinical and Experimental
        Research, 1980, 4, 152-164.

907.   Streissguth, A. P., Martin, D. C., Barr, H. M.,
        and Martin, J. C. Alcohol, nicotine and
        caffeine use in 1529 pregnant women.
        Paper presented at the Western Psychological
        Association Meeting, Seattle, Washington,
        1977.

908.   Streissguth, A. P., Martin, J. C., Martin, D. C.,
        and Barr, H. M. Alcohol and nicotine ingestion
        in pregnant women. Paper presented at the
        Western Psychological Association Meeting,
        Seattle, Washington, 1977.

909.   Strobino, B. R., Kline, J., and Stein, Z.
        Clinical and physical exposures of parents:
        Effects on human reproduction and offspring.
        Early Human Development, 1978, 1, 371-399.

910.   Strudel, G. Action teratogene du sulfate de
        nicotine sur l'embryon de poulet. (Teratogenic
        action of nicotine sulfate on the chick
        embryo.) Comptes Rendus Hebdomadaires des
        Seances de l'Académie des Sciences, 1971, 272,
        673-676.

911.   Strudel, G. and Gateau, G. Étude de l'action
        teratogene du sulfate de nicotine sur les
        stades jeunes de l'embryon de poulet. (Study
        of the teratogenic action of nicotine sulfate
        on the early stages of the chick embryo.)
        Comptes Rendus Hebdomadaires des Seances de
        l'Académie des Sciences, 1971, 272, 2480-
        2483.

912.   Strudel, G. and Gateau, G. Teratogenic action of
        nicotine sulfate on the chick embryo. Tera-
        tology, 1973, 8, 239.

913.   Subak-Sharpe, G.   Is your sex life going up in
            smoke?   Today's Health, 1974, 52, 50-53.

914.   Suematusu, T.   Über den Einfluss des Tabak-
            extraktes auf das Gewebe der innersekretorischen
            Organe. (Concerning the influence of tobacco
            extract on the tissue of inner-secreting
            organs.)   Folia Endocrinologia Japonica,
            1931, 6, 1677-1713.

915.   Suzuki, K., Horiguchi, T., Comas-Urrutia, A. C.,
            Mueller-Heubach, E., Morishima, H. O., and
            Adamsons, K.   Pharmacologic effects of nicotine
            upon the fetus and mother in the rhesus monkey.
            American Journal of Obstetrics and Gynecology,
            1971, 111, 1092-1101.

916.   Suzuki, K., Horiguchi, T., Comas-Urrutia, A. C.,
            Mueller-Heubach, E., Morishima, H. O., and
            Adamsons, K.   Placental transfer and distribution
            of nicotine in the pregnant rhesus monkey.
            American Journal of Obstetrics and Gynecology,
            1974, 119, 253-262.

917.   Suzuki, K., Minei, L. J., and Johnson, E.   Effect
            of nicotine upon uterine blood flow in the
            pregnant rhesus monkey.   American Journal of
            Obstetrics and Gynecology, 1980, 136, 1009-1013.

918.   Sweden, Board of Health Committee.   Concerning
            The Excessive Use of Tobacco and Its Effect
            on the Common People.   Stockholm, 1785.

919.   Sybulski, S.   Umbilical cord plasma cortisol levels
            in association with pregnancy complications.
            Obstetrics and Gynecology, 1977, 50, 308-312.

920.   Szuets, T., Olsson, S., Lindquist, N. G., and
            Ullberg, S.   Long-term fate of ^{14}C-nicotine
            in the mouse: Retention in the bronchi, melanin-
            containing tissues and urinary bladder wall.
            Toxicology, 1978, 10, 207-220.

T

921.   Takeda, M. Influence of some drugs on the action of nicotine
        in chick embryo. Nippon Yakurigaku Zasshi, 1958, 54,
        762-790. (In Japanese.)

922.   Tanaka, M. Smoking and pregnancy. Sanfujinka Chiryo, 1964,
        9, 718-722. (In Japanese.)

923.   Tanaka, M. Studies on the etiological mechanism of fetal
        developmental disorders caused by maternal smoking during
        pregnancy. Nippon Sanka-Fujinka Gakkai Zasshi, 1965, 17,
        1107-1114.

924.   Targett, C. S., Gunesee, H., McBride, F., and Beischer, N. A.
        An evaluation of the effects of smoking on maternal oes-
        triol excretion during pregnancy and on fetal outcome.
        Journal of Obstetrics and Gynaecology of the British
        Commonwealth, 1973, 80, 815-821.

925.   Targett, C. S., Ratten, G. J., Abell, D. A., and Beischer,
        N. A. The influence of smoking on intrauterine fetal
        growth and on maternal oestriol excretion. Australian
        and New Zealand Journal of Obstetrics and Gynaecology,
        1977, 17, 126-130.

926.   Taub, H. J. (editor). Natural Health and Medicine. Pyramid
        Books, New York, 1975.

927.   Tennes, K. and Blackard, C. Maternal alcohol consumption,
        birth weight, and minor physical anomalies. American
        Journal of Obstetrics and Gynecology, 1980, 138, 774-780.

928.   Teraki, Y. Effect of nicotine on development of chicken em-
        bryo with special reference to protein electrophoretic
        pattern in amniotic fluid and allantoic fluid of nico-
        tine hydrops. Teratology, 1976, 14, 258.

929.   Teraki, Y. and Nagumo, K. Effect of nicotine on the develop-
        ment of the chicken embryo, with special reference to its
        relationship with reduced fetal growth, anemia, and res-
        piration. Teratology, 1977, 16, 125.

930.   Terasaka, M. Beitrage zur Pharmakologie des isolierten Uter-
        us. (Studies on the pharmacology of the isolated uter--
        us.) Chosen Igaku Kwai Zasshi, 1927, 81, 749-781.

931.   Terkel, J., Blake, C. A., Hoover, V., and Sawyer, C. H. Pup
        survival and prolactin levels in nicotine-treated lac-
        tating rats. Proceedings of the Society for Experimen-
        tal Biology and Medicine, 1973, 143, 1131-1135.

932.   Terrin, M. and Meyer, M. B. Birth weight-specific rates as
        a bias in the effects of smoking and other perinatal
        hazards. Obstetrics and Gynecology, 1981, 58, 636-638.

933.   Terris, M. and Gold, E. M. An epidemiologic study of pre-
        maturity. American Journal of Obstetrics and Gynecol-
        ogy, 1969, 103, 358-379.

934.   Tescher, M., Rudelin, D., and Maloux, G. Drogues et tabac
        pendant la grossesse. (Drugs and tobacco in pregnancy.)
        Revue du Praticien, 1978, 28, 809-812, 815-816, 819.

935.   Thaler, I., Goodman, J. D. S., and Dawes, G. S. Effects of
        maternal cigarette smoking on fetal breathing and fetal
        movements. American Journal of Obstetrics and Gynecol-
        ogy, 1980, 138, 282-287.

936.   Theberge-Rousselet, D. Babies at risk? Canadian Nurse,
        1976, 72, 34-35.

937.   Thebasius, G. D. Deutliche und ausführliche Nachricht Vom
        Rauch- und Schnupf-Taback worinnen von dessen Nahmen,
        Uhrsprung, Pflanzung, Principiis Chymicis, Wirkungen in
        der Medizin und Chirurgie, vom Rauchen und dessen Miss-
        brauch und erfolgenden Schäden vom Nutzen des Rauchens
        vom wahren und schädlichen Gebrauch des Schnupf-Tabacks
        gehandelt wird: Zur Erhaltung der Gesundheit vorge-
        stellt. (Clear and Thorough Account of Smoking- and
        Snuff-Tobacco Wherein Are Considered Its Names, Origin,
        Cultivation, Chemical Principles, Effects in Medicine
        and Surgery, Smoking and Its Ensuing Evils, Proper and
        Injurious Use of Snuff-Tobacco. Presented for the Pre-
        servation of Health.) Christoph Andreas Zeitler, Uni-
        versity Printer, Halle, 1713.

938.   Thienes, C. H. Failure of nicotine to alter the estrus cycle
        in the white rat. Proceedings of the Society for Exper-
        imental Biology and Medicine, 1931, 28, 740-741.

939.   Thienes, C. H. Chronic nicotine poisoning. Annals of the
        New York Academy of Sciences, 1960, 90, 239-248.

940.   Thienes, C. H., Lombard, C. F., Fielding, F. J., Lesser,
        A. J., and Ellenhorn, M. J. Alterations in reproductive
        functions of white rats associated with daily exposure
        to nicotine. Journal of Pharmacology and Experimental
        Therapeutics, 1946, 87, 1-10.

941.   Thienes, C. H., Lombard, C. F., and Lesser, A. J. Effects
        of chronic nicotine poisoning of rats on viability of
        the young and on the adrenal gland. Journal of Pharma-
        cology and Experimental Therapeutics, 1941, 72, 40P.

942.   Thompson, W. B. Nicotine in breast milk. American Journal
        of Obstetrics and Gynecology, 1933, 26, 662-667.

943.   Tjalve, H., Hansson, E., and Schmiterlow, C. G. Passage of
        ^{14}C-nicotine and its metabolites into mice foetuses and
        placentae. Acta Pharmacologica et Toxicologica, 1968,
        26, 539-555.

944.   Tobias, M., Ayromlooi, J., and Desiderio, D. M. Effects of
        nicotine upon the acid-base status and the hemodynamics
        of chronically instrumented pregnant sheep. Pediatric
        Research, 1980, 14, 613.

945.   Tokieda, K. Über die pharmakologische Wirkung des Ergotox-
        ins, inbesondere in Kombination mit anderen Giften.
        (Concerning the pharmacological effects of ergotoxins
        individually and in combination with other agents.)
        Folio Pharmacologica Japon, 1927, 5, 135-166.

946.   Tokuhata, G. Smoking in relation to infertility and fetal
        loss. Archives of Environmental Health, 1968, 17, 353-
        359.

947.   Tokuhata, G. K., Colflesh, V. G., Smith, M. W., and Digion,
        E. Maternal characteristics and pregnancy outcome.
        American Journal of Epidemiology, 1977, 106, 234-235.

948.   Tomatis, L. Prenatal exposure to chemical carcinogens and
        its effect on subsequent generations. National Cancer
        Institute Monographs, 1979, 51, 159-184.

949.   Tonn, O. Ein Beitrag zum Übergang von Arzteinmitteln in die
        Muttermilch. (A contribution to the passage of drugs
        into the mother's milk.) Pharmazeutische Zentralhalle
        für Deutschland, 1932, 73, 727.

950.   Tournade, A., Chevillot, M., and Bernot, E. Sur certains
        troubles due fonctionnement nerveux engendres par l'in-
        halation de fumée de tabac: Suppression momentanée de
        la reflectivité tendineuse et de l'excitabilité des
        nerfs erecteurs. (On certain problems of nervous func-
        tion engendered by the inhalation of tobacco smoke:
        Momentary suppression of the tendon reflex and the ex-
        citability of the erector nerves.) Comptes Rendus des
        Sciences de la Société de Biologie, 1938, 128, 787-789.

951.   Tryon, T. The Way to Health. Andrew Sowle, London, 1683.

952.   Tsafrir, J. and Halbrecht, I. Birth weight in various popu-
        lation groups in Israel. Social Biology, 1973, 20, 71-
        81.

953.   Tsunoo, S. The pharmacology of tobacco. Bulletin of the Showa Medical School, 1958, 17, 481-489. (In Japanese.)

954.   Tsunoo, S., Muto, Y., Karaki, A., Yamada, T., Kiwaki, T., Iwakura, H., Togami, T., Fujinuma, K., Oku, I., Hayashida, H., Fujikawa, H., and Watanabe, M. Pharmacological studies on nicotine: The effect and the toxicity of nicotine on the general development of chick embryos. Bulletin of the Showa Medical School, 1954, 14, 223-245. (In Japanese.)

955.   Tsunoo, S., Takahashi, K., Kato, S., Naganuma, Y., Yafuso, T., Bessho, T., and Kimura, I. Experimental malformation of chick embryo. Nippon Yakungaku Zasshi, 1959, 55, 1051-1060. (In Japanese.)

956.   Tuchmann-Duplessis, H. Drug Effects on the Fetus. Publishing Sciences Group, Acton, Massachusetts, 1975.

957.   Tuchmann-Duplessis, H. Influence of environmental agents on mammalian foetal development. Proceedings of the Royal Society of Medicine, 1968, 61, 1289-1290.

U

958.   Unbehaun, G. Untersuchungen über die Einwirkung
         des Nicotins auf das Ovarius des weissen
         Maus.(Examination of the effects of nicotine
         on the ovary of the white mouse.) Archiv
         fuer Gynäkologie, 1931, 147, 371-383.

959.   Underwood, P., Hester, L. L., Laffitte, T., and
         Gregg, K. V. The relationship of smoking to
         the outcome of pregnancy. American Journal
         of Obstetrics and Gynecology, 1965, 91, 270-
         276.

960.   Underwood, P., Kesler,K. F., O'Lane, J. M., and
         Callagan, D. A. Parental smoking empirically
         related to pregnancy outcome. Obstetrics
         and Gynecology, 1967, 29, 1-8.

961.   United States Public Health Service. Smoking
         and Health. Report of the Advisory Committee
         to the Surgeon General of the Public Health
         Service. Department of Health,Education, and
         Welfare, DHEW Publication No. 1103, Washington,
         D. C., 1964.

962.   United States Public Health Service. The Health
         Consequences of Smoking. A Report of the
         Surgeon General. Department of Health,
         Education, and Welfare, DHEW Publication
         No. (HSM) 71-7513, Washington, D. C., 1971.

963.   United States Public Health Service. The Health
         Consequences of Smoking. A Report of the
         Surgeon General. Department of Health,
         Education, and Welfare, DHEW Publication
         No. (HSM) 72-7516, Washington, D. C., 1972.

964.   United States Public Health Service. The Health Conse-
        quences of Smoking. A Report of the Surgeon General.
        Department of Health, Education, and Welfare. DHEW
        Publication No. (HSM) 73-8704, Washington, D. C.,
        1973.

965.   United States Public Health Service. The Health Conse-
        quences of Smoking. A Report of the Surgeon General.
        Department of Health, Education, and Welfare. DHEW
        Publication No. (CDC) 76-8704, Washington, D. C.,
        1976.

966.   United States Public Health Service. Smoking and Health:
        A Report of the Surgeon General. Department of
        Health, Education, and Welfare. DHEW Publication No.
        (PHS) 79-50066, Washington, D. C., 1979.

966a.   United States Public Health Service. The Health Conse-
        quences of Smoking for Women: A Report of the Sur-
        geon General. U. S. Department of Health and Human
        Services. Office on Smoking and Health, Rockville,
        Md., 1980.

967.   Upshall, D. G. Correlation of chick embryo teratogenicity
        with the nicotinic activity of a series of tetrahydro-
        pyrimidines. Teratology, 1971, 4, 502.

968.   Upshall, D. G. Correlation of chick embryo teratogenicity
        with the nicotinic activity of a series of tetrahydro-
        pyrimidines. Teratology, 1972, 5, 287-294.

969.   Upshall, D. G., Roger, J., and Casida, J. E. Biochemical
        studies on the teratogenic action of bidrin and other
        neuroactive agents in developing hen eggs. Biochem-
        ical Pharmacology, 1968, 17, 1529-1542.

970.   Usher, R. H. and McLean, F. H. Normal fetal growth and
        the significance of fetal growth retardation. In
        Davis, J. A. and Dobbing, J. (editors). Scientific
        Foundations of Paediatrics. William Heinemann Medical
        Books, London, 1974.

V

971. Vaehaekangas, K., Hirn, M., and Pelkonen, O.
      Effect of maternal cigarette smoking decreases
      birthweight. Acta Physiologica Scandinavica,
      1980, Supplement 473, 274.

972. Valdes-Dapena, M. A. Sudden infant death
      syndrome: A review of the medical literature
      1974-1979. Pediatrics, 1980, 66, 597-614.

973. Van den Berg, B. J. Smoking and pregnancy.
      Nature, 1973, 246, 540.

974. Van den Berg, B. J. Epidemiologic observations
      of prematurity: Effects of tobacco, coffee
      and alcohol. In Reed, D. M. and Stanley, F. J.
      (editors). The Epidemiology of Prematurity.
      Urban and Schwarzenberg, Munich, 1977,
      157-176.

975. Vangen, O. Rokevaner hos gravide kvinner i
      hedmark. (Smoking habits among pregnant women
      in Hedmark.) Tidsskrift for den Norske
      Laegeforening, 1974, 96, 639-641.

976. Van Hoosen, B. Should women smoke? Motherhood
      and tobacco antagonistic. Medical Women's
      Journal, 1952, 34, 226-227.

977. Van Keep, P. A., Brand, P. C., and Lehert, P.
      Factors affecting the age at menopause.
      Journal of Biosocial Science, 1979, 6
      (Supplement), 37-55.

978. Van Vunakis, H., Langone, J. J., and Milunsky, A.
      Nicotine and cotinine in the amniotic fluid
      of smokers in the second trimester of pregnancy.
      American Journal of Obstetrics and Gynecology,
      1974, 120, 64-66.

979.   Vara, P. and Kinnunen, O. The effect of nicotine
        on the female rabbit and developing fetus.
        Annales Medicinae Experimentales et Biologiae
        Fenniae, 1951, 29, 202-213.

980.   Vaught, J. B., Gurtoo, H. L., Parker, N. B.,
        Leboeuf, R., and Doctor, G. Effects of smoking
        on benzo(a)pyrene metabolism by human placental
        microsomes. Cancer Research, 1979, 39,
        3177-3183.

981.   Vavercak, F. Smoking and pregnancy. Ceskoslo-
        venska Gynekologie, 1968, 33, 197-200.

982.   Venulet, F. and Danysz, A. Wpływ dymu tytoniowego
        na poziom kwasu askorbinowego w mleku kobiecym.
        (The effect of tobacco smoke on ascorbic
        acid in human milk.) Acta Physiologica
        Polonica, 1954, 4, 646.

983.   Venulet, F. and Danysz, A. Wpływ palenia tytoniu
        na poziom witaminy c mleku kobiecym. (Influence
        of tobacco smoke on vitamin C content in
        mother's milk.) Pediatria Polska, 1955,
        30, 811-817.

984.   Vértes, L. Schädliche Wirkungen vom Rauchen auf
        die Gestation. (Noxious effects of smoking
        on gestation.) Zentralblatt für Gynäkologie,
        1970, 92, 1395-1398.

985.   Vessey, M., Meisler, L., Flavel, R., and Yeates, D.
        Outcome of pregnancy in women using different
        methods of contraception. British Journal
        of Obstetrics and Gynecology, 1979, 86, 548-
        556.

986.   Viczián, M. Dohányosokon végzett ondóvizsgálatok
        tapasztalatai. (Experiences with the
        sperm of smokers.) Orvosi Hetilap, 1968,
        109, 1077-1079.

987.   Viczián, M. The effect of cigarette smoke inhal-
        ation on spermatogenesis in rat. Experientia,
        1968, 24, 511-512.

988.   Viczián, M. Ergebnisse von Spermauntersuchungen
        bie Zigarettenrauchern. (Results of spermatozoa
        studies in cigarette smokers.) Zeitschrift
        fuer Haut und Geschlechts-Krankheiten, 1969,
        44, 183-187.

989.   Villani, C. and Mazzon, I. Smoking in pregnancy.
        Effect on gestation and consequent effects on
        the fetus. Minerva Ginecologia 1981, 33,
        117-126.

990.   Villumsen, A. L.   Cigarette smoking and low birth weight.
        Ugeskrift for Laegeforening, 1962, 124, 630-631.

991.   Villumsen, A. L.   Environmental factors and congenital
        malformations. Teratology, 1971, 4, 503.

992.   Von Criegern, T.   Smoking and alcohol consumption in
        pregnancy: A subtle form of child abuse.   Schwestern
        Revue, 1979, 17, 19-20.

993.   Von Hofstatter, R.   Experimentelle Studie über die Ein-
        wirkung des Nikotins auf die Keimdrusen und auf die
        Fortpflanzung. (Experimental studies on the effects
        of nicotine on the gonads and on propogation.)
        Virchows Archiv Abteilung. A. Pathologische Anatomie
        und Physiologie, 1923, 244, 183-213.

994.   Von Stammler, M.   Nikotin und Nebennieren. (Nicotine
        and adrenals.)   Deutsche Medizinische Wochenschrift,
        1932, 1, 1960-1963.

995.   Von Stammler, M.   Die chronische Vergiftung mit Nikotin.
        (Chronic poisoning with nicotine.)   Virchows Archiv
        Abteilung. A. Pathologische Anatomie und Physiologie,
        1935, 295, 366-393.

996.   Von Stammler, M.   Nikotin und Keimdrusen. (Nicotine and
        the gonads.)   Münchener Medizinische Wochenschrift,
        1936, 83, 658.

997.   Vorherr, H.   Drug excretion in breast milk.   Post-
        graduate Medicine, 1974, 56, 97-104.

998.   Vuori, E., Tylinen, H., Kuitunen, P., and Paganus, A.
        The occurrence and origin of DDT in human milk.
        Acta Paediatrica Scandinavica, 1977, 66, 761-765.

999.   Waddell, J. A.   The pharmacology of the vas deferens.
        Journal of Pharmacology and Experimental Therapeutics,
        1916, 8, 551-559.

1000.   Waddell, J. A.   The pharmacology of the seminal ves-
        icles.   Journal of Pharmacology and Experimental
        Therapeutics, 1917, 9, 113-120.

1001.   Waddell, J. A.   The pharmacology of the uterus mascu-
        linus.   Journal of Pharmacology and Experimental
        Therapeutics, 1917, 9, 171-178.

1002.   Waddell, J. A.   The pharmacology of the vagina.
        Journal of Pharmacology and Experimental Therapeutics,
        1917, 9, 411-426.

1003.   Waddell, W. J. and Marlowe, G. C.   Whole-body auto-
        radiography of the distribution of nicotine-14C in
        pregnant mice.   Teratology, 1973, 7, 29A-30A.

1004.   Waddell, W. J. and Marlowe, G. C.   Localization of
        nicotine-14C, cotinine-14C, and nicotine-1'-N-oxide-
        14C in tissues of the mouse.   Drug Metabolism and
        Disposition, 1976, 4, 530-539.

1005.   Wagner, B., Lazar, P., and Chouroulinkov, I.   The
        effects of cigarette smoke inhalation upon mice
        during pregnancy.   Revue Europeene d'Études Cliniques
        et Biologiques, 1972, 17, 943-948.

1006.   Wang, I. Y., Rasmussen, R. E., Creasey, R., and
        Crocker, T. T.   Metabolites of benzo(a)pyrene pro-
        duced by placental microsomes from cigarette
        smokers and nonsmokers.   Life Sciences, 1977, 20,
        1265-1272.

1007.   Weathersbee, P. S. Nicotine and its influence on the
         female reproductive system. Journal of Reproductive
         Medicine, 1980, 25, 243-250.

1008.   Weathersbee, P. S. and Lodge, J. R. Alcohol, caffeine,
         and nicotine as factors in pregnancy. Postgraduate
         Medicine, 1979, 66, 165-167, 170-171.

1009.   Welch, R. M., Gommi, B., Alvares, A., and Conney, A. H.
         Effect of enzyme induction on the metabolism of
         benzo(a)pyrene and 3-methyl-4-monomethylaminoazo-
         benzene in the pregnant and fetal rat. Cancer Re-
         search, 1972, 32, 973-978.

1010.   Welch, R. M., Harrison, Y. E., Conney, A. H., Poppers,
         P. J., and Finster, M. Cigarette smoking: Stimula-
         tory effect on metabolism of 3,4 benzpyrene by enzymes
         in human placenta. Science, 1968, 160, 541-542.

1011.   Wellband, W. A., Miner, N., and Steinhaus, A. H. Effect
         of tobacco smoke on the artificially induced vaginal
         cycle in spayed rats. Federation Proceedings, 1957,
         16, 136.

1012.   Wenderlein, J. M. Rauchen und Schwangerschaft: Psycho-
         soziale Aspekte zur Pravention von Nikotinschaden.
         (Smoking and pregnancy: Psychosocial aspects of pre-
         vention from nicotine-induced damage.) Zeitschrift
         für Geburtshilfe Perinatologie, 1977, 181, 368-375.

1013.   Wenger, B. S. and Wenger, E. L. Nicotine as a be-
         havioral teratogen. Anatomical Record, 1977, 187,
         746.

1014.   Wennerberg, P. A. and Welsch, F. Effects of cholinergic
         drugs on uptake of 14-C-amminoisobutyric acid by
         human term placenta fragments: Implication for acetyl-
         choline recognition sites and observations on the
         binding of radioactive cholinergic ligands. Feder-
         ation Proceedings, 1977, 36, 980.

1015.   West, S., Matanoski, G., and Gordis, L. Occupation
         and environmental exposures and the risk of congenital
         heart defects. American Journal of Epidemiology,
         1980, 112, 446.

1016.   Whelan, E. M., Sheridan, M. J., Meister, K. A., and
         Mosher, B. A. Analysis of coverage of tobacco
         hazards in women's magazines. Journal of Public
         Health Policy, 1981, 2, 28-35.

1017.   Whichelow, M. J. Breast feeding in Cambridge, England:
         Factors affecting the mother's milk supply. Journal
         of Advanced Nursing, 1979, 4, 253-261.

1018.   Whichelow, M. J. and King, B. E. Breast feeding and
         smoking. Archives of Diseases of Children, 1979,
         54, 240-245.

1019.   Whitelaw, A. G. L. Influence of maternal obesity on
         subcutaneous fat in the newborn. British Medical
         Journal, 1976, 1, 985-986.

1020.   Wilcox, A. J. Birth weight, gestation, and the fetal
         growth curve. American Journal of Obstetrics and
         Gynecology, 1981, 139, 863-867.

1021.   Willenbrecher, T. Why the Turk can't get it up.
         Mother Jones, 1979, 4, 37-38.

1022.   Williams, H. S. and Meyer, M. B. Cigarette smoking,
         infant birth weight, and perinatal mortality rates.
         American Journal of Obstetrics and Gynecology, 1973,
         116, 890-892.

1023.   Williams, H. S. and Meyer, M. B. Cigarette smoking,
         infant birth weight, and perinatal mortality. Reply
         to Dr. Yerushalmy. American Journal of Obstetrics
         and Gynecology, 1974, 118, 886-888.

1024.   Willson, J. R. The effect of nicotine on lactation in
         white mice. American Journal of Obstetrics and
         Gynecology, 1942, 43, 839-844.

1025.   Wilson, E. W. The effect of smoking in pregnancy on
         the placental coefficient. New Zealand Medical
         Journal, 1972, 74, 384-385.

1026.   Wilson, R. H. and De Eds, F. Nicotine toxicity.
         III. Effect of nicotine-containing diets on the
         estrus cycle. Journal of Pharmacology and Exper-
         imental Therapeutics, 1937, 59, 260-263.

1027.   Wilson, R. H., McNaught, J. B., and De Eds, F.
         Chronic nicotine toxicity. IV. Effect of nicotine-
         containing diets on histology and weights of organs
         of albino rats. Journal of Industrial Hygiene and
         Toxicology, 1938, 20, 468-481.

1028.   Wingerd, J., Christianson, R., Lovitt, W. V., and
         Schoen, E. J. Placental ratio in white and black
         women: Relation to smoking and anemia. American
         Journal of Obstetrics and Gynecology, 1976, 124,
         671-675.

1029.   Wingerd, J. and Schoen, E. J. Factors influencing
         length at birth and height at five years. Pediatrics,
         1974, 53, 737-741.

1030.   Winkelstein, W. Smoking and cancer of the uterine
         cervix: Hypothesis. American Journal of Epidemiology,
         1977, 106, 257-259.

1031.   Winter, R. Hormones and tobacco smoke--When mixed it's
         all ill wind. Science Digest, 1980, 88, 58-61.

1032.   Winternitz, W. W. and Quillen, D. Acute hormonal re-
         sponse to cigarette smoking. Journal of Clinical
         Pharmacology, 1977, 17, 389-397.

1033.   Witte, J. J. The hazards of cigarette smoking during
         pregnancy. Journal of the Maine Medical Association,
         1978, 69, 314, 316, 320.

1034.   Witte, J. J. Effects of cigarette smoking during
         pregnancy. Journal of the Medical Association of
         Georgia, 1979, 68, 386-388.

1035.   Witter, F. and King, T. M. Cigarettes and pregnancy.
         In Schwarz, R. H. and Yaffe, S. J. (editors). Drug
         and Chemical Risks to the Fetus and Newborn.
         Alan R. Liss, New York, 1980, 83-92.

1036.   Wolman, I. J. When a mother smokes during pregnancy,
         will it affect her baby? Clinical Pediatrics, 1974,
         13, 485-486.

1037.   Wood, A. J. Smoking and pregnancy. Nursing Mirror.
         1973, 137, 26-28.

1038.   Wood, C. Gynaecological survey in a metropolitan area
         of Melbourne. Australian and New Zealand Journal
         of Obstetrics and Gynaecology, 1972, 12, 147-156.

1039.   Wood, C. The association of psycho-social factors and
         gynaecological symptoms. Australian Family Physician,
         1978, 7, 471, 473, 475, 477-478.

1040.   Wood, C., Gilbert, M., O'Connor, A., and Walters, W. A. W.
         Subjective recording of fetal movement. British
         Journal of Obstetrics and Gynecology, 1979, 86, 838-
         842.

1041.   Wood, C., Larsen, L., and Williams, R. Duration of
         menstruation. Australian and New Zealand Journal of
         Obstetrics and Gynaecology, 1979, 19, 216-229.

1042.   Wood, C., Larsen, L., and Williams, R. Social and
         psychological factors in relation to premenstrual
         tension and menstrual pain. Australian and New Zea-
         land Journal of Obstetrics and Gynaecology, 1979,
         19, 111-115.

1043.   World Health Organization. Smoking and disease:
         The evidence reviewed. WHO Chronicle, 1975, 29,
         402-408.

1044.   World Health Organization. Smoking and Its Effects on
         Health. Report of a WHO Expert Committee. WHO
         Technical Report Series, 568. World Health Organ-
         ization, Geneva, 1975.

1045.   World Health Organization. Gestation, birth-weight,
         and spontaneous abortion in pregnancy after induced
         abortion. Report of collaborative study by W.H.O.
         task force on sequelae of abortion. Lancet, 1979,
         1, 142-145.

1046.   Wright, S. Some results of experiments on the physio-
         logical action of tobacco. London Medical Gazette,
         1846, 92, 592-593.

1047.   Wynder, E. L. and Hoffmann, D. Tobacco and health:
         A societal challenge. New England Journal of
         Medicine, 1979, 300, 894-903.

Y

1048. Yaffe, S. J. A clinical look at the problem of drugs
       in pregnancy and their effect on the fetus. Canadian
       Medical Association Journal, 1975, 112, 728-733.

1049. Yamasaki, E. and Ames, B. N. Concentration of mutagens
       from urine by adsorption with the nonpolar resin
       XAD-2: Cigarette smokers have mutagenic urine.
       Proceedings of the National Academy of Sciences,
       1977, 74, 3555-3559.

1050. Yerushalmy, J. Mother's cigarette smoking and survival
       of infant. American Journal of Obstetrics and
       Gynecology, 1964, 88, 505-518.

1051. Yerushalmy, J. Cigarette smoking and infant survival.
       American Journal of Obstetrics and Gynecology, 1965,
       91, 881.

1052. Yerushalmy, J. On inferring causality from observed
       associations. In Ingelfinger, F. J., Relman, A. S.,
       and Finland, M. (editors). Controversy in Internal
       Medicine. W. B. Saunders, Philadelphia, 1966, 659-668.

1053. Yerushalmy, J. The relationship of parents' cigarette
       smoking to outcome of pregnancy--Implications as to
       the problem of inferring causation from observed
       associations. American Journal of Epidemiology, 1971,
       93, 443-456.

1054. Yerushalmy, J. Birthweight and the displacement hypo-
       thesis. American Journal of Epidemiology, 1972, 95,
       2.

1055. Yerushalmy, J. Cigarette smoking and low-birth weight
       babies. Reply to Mr. Goldstein. American Journal
       of Obstetrics and Gynecology, 1972, 114, 571-573.

1056.   Yerushalmy, J. Infants with low birth weight born before
         their mothers started to smoke cigarettes. American
         Journal of Obstetrics and Gynecology, 1972, 112, 277-
         284.

1057.   Yerushalmy, J. Self-selection--A major problem in
         observational studies. In LeCam, L. N., Neyman, J.,
         and Scott, E. L. (editors). Proceedings of the Sixty
         Berkeley Symposium on Mathematical Statistics and
         Probability. University of California Press, Berkeley,
         California, 1972, 329-342.

1058.   Yerushalmy, J. Congenital heart disease and maternal
         smoking habits. Nature, 1973, 242, 262.

1059.   Yerushalmy, J. Smoking in pregnancy. Developmental
         Medicine and Child Neurology, 1973, 15, 691.

1060.   Yerushalmy, J. The cigarette controversy. Congressional
         Record--Senate, 1973, February 7, S2342-S2343.

1061.   Yerushalmy, J. Cigarette smoking, infant birth weight
         and perinatal mortality rates. American Journal of
         Obstetrics and Gynecology, 1974, 118, 884-886.

1062.   Yeung, D. L., Pennell, M. D., Leung, M., and Hall, J.
         Breastfeeding: Prevalence and influencing factors.
         Canadian Journal of Public Health, 1981, 72, 323-330.

1063.   Yeung, D. L., Pennell, M. D., Leung, M., and Hall, J.
         Effects of maternal cigarette smoking during preg-
         nancy on birthsize, growth of infants and infant
         feeding practices. Nutrition Reports International,
         1981, 23, 887-900.

1064.   Yeung, K. R. Smoking in pregnancy. British Medical
         Journal, 1981, 282, 2057.

1065.   Yoshinaga, K., Rice, C., Krenn, J., and Pilot, R. L.
         Effects of nicotine on early pregnancy in the rat.
         Biology of Reproduction, 1979, 20, 294-303.

1066.   Young, I. M. and Pugh, L. G. E. The carbon monozide
         content of fetal and maternal blood. Journal of
         Obstetrics and Gynecology of the British Commonwealth,
         1963, 70, 681.

1067.   Younoszai, M. K. Effect of maternal smoking on hemo-
         globin and hematocrit of the newborn. American
         Journal of Clinical Nutrition, 1979, 32, 1983.

1068.   Younoszai, M. K., Kacid, A., and Haworth, J. C.
         Cigarette smoking during pregnancy: The effect
         upon the haematocrit and acid-base balance of the
         newborn infant. Canadian Medical Association Jour-
         nal, 1968, 99, 197-200.

1069.   Younoszai, M. K., Peloso, J., and Haworth, J. C. Fetal
         growth retardation in rats exposed to cigarette
         smoke during pregnancy. American Journal of Obstet-
         rics and Gynecology, 1969, 104, 1207-1213.

Z

1070.   Zabriskie, J. R. Effect of cigarette smoking during pregnancy. *Obstetrics and Gynecology*, 1963, 21, 405-411.

1071.   Zenk, K. E. An overview of perinatal clinical pharmacology. *Clinics in Laboratory Medicine*, 1981, 1, 361-375.

Addendum

A

1072. Abdul-Karim, R. W. and Beydoun, S. N. Growth of the human fetus. _Clinical Obstetrics and Gynecology_, 1974, _17_, 37-52.

1073. Adler, I. Preliminary note on some effects of tobacco on the tissues of rabbits. _Journal of Medical Research_, 1902, _8_, 309-315.

1074. Afanassiev, K. M. Effects of nicotine on the sexual function of man. _Vrachebnaia Gazeta_, 1931, _35_, 1617-1619.

1075. Affaitati, **C.** _Il semplice ortolano in villa, e l'accurato giardiniere in città, cioè regole pratiche, e fondate su l'esperienza di vecchj ortolani, per coltivare qualunque sorte d'erbaggi per propagare, innestare piante, viti, ec. Trattato del tobacco, avvisi per la economia, cura de' mori, e bigatti. Regole per la coltura de' fiori, e governo degli agrumi._ (The simple gardener in the villa, and the accurate gardener in the city, i.e., practical rules, founded on the experience of old gardeners, for cultivating whatever sort of pot-herbs, for propagating and grafting plants, vines, etc. Treatise on tobacco, advice on the economy and care of mulberry trees and silkworms. Rules for cultivating flowers, and treating pot-herbs.) Federigo Agnelli, Milan, 1758.

1076. Agar, W. T. The action of adrenaline upon the uterus of the guinea pig and its modification by eserine. _Journal of Physiology_, 1940, _98_, 492-502.

1077. Akkermann, S., Grindel, B.; and Seidenschnur, G. Zur Epidemiologie der Frühgeburtlichkeit Berufstätiger. (Epidemiology of premature birth in women who work.) _Zentralblatt für Gynäkologie_, 1978, _100_, 1153-1161.

1078.   Alaverdian, A. G., Kalantarova, L. G., Arakelian, R. N.,
         and Kazarian, L. G. Morphological changes in the uter-
         us and placenta of pregnant rats under the influence
         of tobacco smoke. Zhurnal Exsperimental'noi i Klin-
         icheskoi Meditsiny, 1976, 16, 37-43. (In Russian.)

1079.   Alaverdian, A. G., Kalantarova, L. G., Eshchutkin, G. D.,
         Kirakosian, S. A., and Vanetsian, A. Morphological
         changes in the ovaries, adrenals and pituitary of
         pregnant rats exposed to tobacco smoke chronically.
         Zhurnal Eksperimental'noi i Klinicheskoi Meditsiny,
         1976, 16, 48-52. (In Russian.)

1080.   Alberman, E. D. and Goldstein, H. Possible teratogenic
         effect of cigarette smoking. Nature, 1971, 231, 529-
         539.

1081.   Alexander, J. C., Silverman, N. A., and Chretien, P. B.
         Effect of age and cigarette smoking on carcinoembry-
         onic antigen levels. Journal of the American Medical
         Association, 1976, 235, 1975-1979.

1082.   Alvear, J. and Brooke, O. G. Fetal growth in different
         racial groups. Archives of Diseases of Childhood,
         1978, 53, 27-32.

1083.   Ambrose, A. M. and De Eds, F. Some comparative obser-
         vations on l-nicotine and myosmine. Proceedings of
         the Society for Experimental Biology of New York,
         1946, 63, 423-424.

1084.   American College of Obstetrics and Gynecology.
         Cigarette Smoking and Pregnancy. American College of
         Obstetrics and Gynecology, 1979, Technical Bulletin
         No. 53.

1085.   Amyot, G. Les soins prenataux. (Prenatal care.) Union
         Médicale du Canada, 1975, 104, 1514-1517.

1085a.   Andressen, B. D., Ng, K. J., Iams, J. D., and Bianchine,
         J. R. Cotinine in amniotic fluids from passive
         smokers. Lancet, 1982, 1, 791.

1086.   Andrews, J. Smoking in pregnancy. Midwife and Health
         Visitor, 1972, 8, 239-243.

1087.   Annis, L. F. The Child Before Birth. Cornell University
         Press, Ithaca, New York, 1978.

1088.   Anonymous. Smoking during pregnancy. Time, 1962, 80, 59.

1089.   Anonymous. Mother and baby. Food and Cosmetics Toxicol-
         ogy, 1963, 1, 258-259.

1090.   Anonymous. Lead accumulation in mothers who smoke and
         their fetuses. Public Health Reports, 1977, 92, 491-
         492.

1091.   Anonymous. Best care for babies. Lancet, 1978, 2, 355-
         356.

1092.   Anonymous. Cigarette smoking and spontaneous abortion.
         British Medical Journal, 1978, 1, 259-260.

1093.   Anonymous.   Pill brochure stresses smoking warning.
         FDA Consumer, 1978, 12, 3-4.

1094.   Anonymous. Placental defects linked to smoking. Medical
         World News, 1978, 19, 24, 26.

1095.   Anonymous. Even a late break from smoking could help
         fetus. Medical World News, 1979, 20, 48-49.

1096.   Anonymous. Smoking and intrauterine growth. Lancet,
         1979, 1, 536-537.

1097.   Anonymous. Smoking and pregnancy. Family Health, 1979,
         11, May, 8.

1098.   Anonymous. Smoking hazards and the fetus. Science News,
         1979, 116, 138.

1099.   Anonymous. Smoking imperils the unborn. Science News,
         1979, 115, 55.

1100.   Anonymous. Smoking and sperm. Science News, 1981, 119,
         247.

1101.   Anonymous. When mom smokes, umbilical cells shrivel.
         Medical World News, 1981, 22, 37-38.

1102.   Apgar, V. and Beck, J. Is My Baby All Right? Pocket
         Books, New York, 1974.

1103.   Ardito, G., Lamberti, L., Ansaldi, E., and Ponzetto, P.
         Sister-chromatid exchanges in cigarette-smoking human
         females and their newborns. Mutation Research, 1980,
         78, 209-212.

1104.   Arena, J. M. Contamination of the ideal food. Nutrition
         Today, 1970, 5, 2-8.

1105.   Asmussen, I. Effects of maternal smoking on the fetal
         cardiovascular system. Cardiovascular Medicine, 1979,
         4, 777-790.

1106.   Asmussen, I. Ultrastructure of the villi and fetal
         capillaries in placentas from smoking and nonsmoking
         mothers. British Journal of Obstetrics and Gynecology,
         1980, 87, 239-245.

1107.   Astrup, P., Trolle, D., Olsen, H. M., and Kjeldsen, K.
           Effect of moderate carbon-monoxide exposure on fetal
           development. Lancet, 1972, 2, 1220-1222.

1107a.   Athayde, E. Incidencia de abortos e mortinataldidade
           nas operarias da industria de fumo. (Incidence of
           abortion and neonatal mortality among workers in the
           tobacco industry.) Brasil Medicina, 1948, 62, 237-
           239.

B

1108.   Bacon, F. *Sylva Sylvarum*. William Lee, London, 1626.

1109.   Baer, D. S. Treatment of female mice with tobacco smoke:
        Effects on fertility, maternal care, and offspring
        behavior. Ph.D. Thesis, University of Colorado,
        Boulder, Colorado, 1980.

1110.   Ball, K. P., Andrews, J., Hytten, F. E., Kelnar, C. J. H.,
        and Ross, E. M. Mothers who smoke and their children.
        Practitioner, 1980, 24, 735-740.

1111.   Ballantyne, J. W. *Manual of Antenatal Pathology and
        Hygiene: The Fetus*. William Green and Sons, Edin-
        burgh, 1902.

1112.   Barrett, J. M., Vanhooydonk, J. E., and Boehm, F. H.
        Acute effect of cigarette smoking on the fetal heart
        rate nonstress test. *Obstetrics and Gynecology*, 1981,
        57, 422-425.

1113.   Beal, V. A. Nutritional studies during pregnancy. *Jour-
        nal of the American Dietetic Association*, 1971, 58,
        321-326.

1114.   Beintema van Peima, I. I. W. *Tabacologia, Ofte Korte
        Verhandelenge Over de Tabak, Desselus Deugd, Gebruyk,
        Ende Kennisse: Waar Door Aangeweesen Wordt een Wegh
        om Lang, Vroolijk, Ende Gesond te Leeven*. (Tabacologia,
        or Short Treatise on Tobacco, along with the Virtue,
        Use, and Knowledge of It: In Which [Treatise] Is
        Demonstrated the Way to Live Long, Happily, and
        Healthily.) Levyn van Dyck, The Hague, 1690.

1115.   Berkowitz, G. S. An epidemiologic study of preterm de-
        livery. *American Journal of Epidemiology*, 1981, 113,
        81-92.

1116.   Berlin, C. M. The excretion of drugs in human milk. In
         Schwarz, R. H. and Yaffe, S. J. (editors). Drugs and
         Chemical Risks to the Fetus and Newborn. Alan R. Liss,
         New York, 1980, 115-127.

1117.   Bessho, T. Malformations induced by nornicotine in chick
         embryo. Nippon Yakurigaku Zasshi, 1960, 56, 1223-1224.
         (In Japanese.)

1118.   Betts, C. A. Smokers seek masculinity. Science News Let-
         ter, 1965, 87, 373.

1118a.   Bignami, G. Pharmacologic influences on mating behavior in
         the male rat: Effects of d-amphetamine, LSD-25, strych-
         nine, nicotine and various anticholinergic agents.
         Psychopharmacologica, 1966, 10, 44-58.

1119.   Bjoro, K. Etiologi og klinikk ved intrauterin vekstretard-
         asjon og truende fosterdod. (Etiology and clinical ef-
         fects in intrauterine growth retardation and threat of
         embryonic death.) Tidsskrift for den Norske Laegefor-
         ening, 1972, 92, 1919-1922.

1120.   Black, P. M. The child at risk--Interprofessional co-
         operation. Nursing Mirror, 1977, April, 56-61.

1121.   Bloch, I. The Sexual Life of Our Time in Its Relation to
         Modern Civilization. Allied Book Co., New York, 1928.

1122.   Bodendorfer, T. W., Briggs, G. G., and Gunning, J. E. Ob-
         taining drug exposure histories during pregnancy. Amer-
         ican Journal of Obstetrics and Gynecology, 1979, 135,
         490-494.

1123.   Bogdan, D. P. and Juchau, M. R. Characteristics of induced
         benzpyrene hydroxylase activity in the rat foetoplacen-
         tal unit. European Journal of Pharmacology, 1970, 10,
         119-126.

1124.   Bontekoe, C. Kurze Abhandlung von dem Menschlichen Leben,
         Gesundheit, Kranckheit und Tod in Drey unterschiedenen
         Theilen verfasset, davon das I. Unterricht giebet von
         dem Leibe und desselben zur Gesundheit dienlichen Ver-
         richtungen. II. Von der Kranckheit und derselben Ur-
         sachen. III. Von denen Mitteln das Leben und die Ge-
         sundheit zu unterhalten und zu verlangern die meisten
         Kranckheite aber und ein daraus entstehendes beschwer-
         liches Alter durch Speise, Tranck, Schlaffen, Thee, Cof-
         fee, Chocolate, Taback und andere dergleichen zur Ge-
         sundheit dienliche Mittel eine geraume Zeit zu verhuten.
         Wobey noch angehanget Drey kleine Tractätlein: I. Von
         der Natur. II. Von der Experienz oder Erfahrung.
         III. Von der Gewissheit der Medicin, oder Heil-Kunst.
         (Short Treatise on Human Life, Health, Sickness, and
         Death, Composed in Three Distinct Parts, of Which the
         First Offers Information on the Body and Serviceable

Arrangements for Its Health; the Second, on Sickness
and Its Causes; the Third, on Which Means Life and
Health Is to Be Conserved and Prolonged to Prevent for
a Considerable Time Most Illnesses and Accompanying
Infirmities of Age Stemming from Them Through Proper
Use of Food, Drink, Sleep, Tea, Coffee, Chocolate,
Tobacco, and Other Similar Serviceable Means for
Health. To Which Are Added Three Small Tracts. I. Of
Nature. II. Of Experience or Knowledge. III. Of the
Certainty of Medicine or the Art of Healing.) Fried-
rich Arnsts Publisher, Budissin, 1685.

1125.   Borlée, I., Bouckaert, A., Lechat, M. F., and Mission,
C. B. Smoking patterns during and before pregnancy:
Weight, length and head circumference of progeny.
European Journal of Obstetrics, Gynecology, and Repro-
ductive Biology, 1978, 8, 171-177.

1126.   Borlée, I. and Lechat, M. F. Resultats d'une enquête sur
les malformations congenitales dans le Hainaut. (Results of a study on congenital malformations in
Hainaut.) Archives Belges de Médicine Sociale, Hygiene, Médicine du Travail et Médicine Legale, 1978,
36, 77-99.

1127.   Bosley, A. R. J., Sibert, J. R., and Newcombe, R. G.
Effects of maternal smoking on fetal growth and nutrition. Archives of the Disabled Child, 1981, 56,
727-729.

1128.   Boyce, A., Schwartz, D., and David, G. Smoking and
genitourinary infection. British Medical Journal,
1976, 2, 1013.

1129.   Bracken, M. B. and Holford, T. R. Induced abortion and
congenital malformations in offspring of subsequent
pregnancies. American Journal of Epidemiology, 1979,
109, 425-432.

1130.   Bracken, M. B. and Holford, T. R. Exposure to prescribed
drugs in pregnancy and association with congenital
malformations. Obstetrics and Gynecology, 1981, 58,
336-344.

1131.   Bradt, P. T. and Herrenkohl, R. C. DDT in human milk:
What determines the levels? Science of the Total
Environment, 1976, 6, 161-163.

1132.   Brailsford, E. An Experimental Dissertation on the Chemical and Medical Properties of the Nicotiana Tabacum
of Linnaeus, Commonly Known by the Name of Tobacco.
John Ormrod, Philadelphia, 1799.

1133.   Breart, G., Hennequin, J. F., Crost-Deniel, M., and
           Rumeau-Rouquette, C. Étude de l'insuffisance ponder-
           ale à la naissance. À partir d'un enchantillon repre-
           sentatiff de nouveau-nés. (A study of insufficient
           weight at birth. From a representative sample of
           newborns.) Archives Françaises de Pédiatrie, 1977,
           34 (Supplement 2), 221-232.

1134.   Brent, R. L. and Harris, M. I. (editors). Prevention of
           Embryonic, Fetal, and Perinatal Disease. National
           Institute of Health, Washington, D. C., 1976.

1135.   Brewer, G. S. (editor). The Pregnancy After 30 Workbook.
           Rodale Press, Emmaus, Pennsylvania, 1978.

1136.   Brewer, G. S. and Brewer, T. What Every Pregnant Woman
           Should Know. Random House, New York, 1977.

1137.   Broman, S. H., Nichols, P. L., and Kennedy, W. A. Pre-
           school IQ: Prenatal and Early Development Correlates.
           Lawrence Erlbaum Associates, Hillsdale, New Jersey,
           1975.

1138.   Brooks, J. E. Tobacco, Its History Illustrated by the
           Books, Manuscripts and Engravings in the Library of
           George Arents, Jr., Together with an Introductory
           Essay, a Glossary, and Bibliographic Notes. Vol-
           ume 1: 1507-1615. The Rosenbach Company, New York,
           1937.

1139.   Buchet, J. P., Roels, H., Hubermont, G., and Lauwerys, R.
           Placental transfer of lead, mercury, cadmium, and
           carbon monoxide in women. II. Influence of some epi-
           demiological factors on the frequency distributions
           of the biological indices in maternal and umbilical
           cord blood. Environmental Research, 1978, 15, 494-
           503.

1140.   Bureau, M. A., Monette, J., Pare, C., Lippe, J., Mathieu,
           J. L., Blouin, D., Berthiaume, Y., Begin, R., and
           Shapcott, D. Foetus, fumeur involontaire: Étude du
           monoxyde de carbone chez les femmes enceintes et les
           nouveaunes. (Passive smoking and the fetus: A study
           of carbon monoxide in pregnant women and neonates.)
           Union Médicale du Canada, 1980, 109, 1341-1345.

1141.   Bureau, M. A., Monette, J., Shapcott, D., Pare, C.,
           Mathieu, J. L., Lippe, J., Blovin, D., Berthiaume, Y.,
           and Begin, R. Carboxyhemoglobin concentration in
           fetal cord blood and in blood of mothers who smoked
           during labor. Pediatrics, 1982, 69, 371-373.

1142.   Burn, J. H. Excretion of drugs in milk. British Medical
           Journal, 1947, 5, 1113-1115.

1143.   Burrow, G. N. and Ferris, T. F. Medical Complications
         During Pregnancy. W. B. Saunders Co., Philadelphia,
         Pennsylvania, 1975.

1144.   Bush, P. J. Drugs, Alcohol and Sex. Richard Marek Pub-
         lishers, New York, 1980.

1145.   Bystrom, G., Lungren, M., Meyer-Lie, A., and Palmborg, M.
         En studie over orsaker till missbildningsbord och
         perinatal dodlighet iv Varmland. (A study of factors
         causing birth defects and perinatal mortality in
         Varmland.) Läkartidningen, 1977, 74, 3167-3169.

C

1146.   Cahen, R. L. Evaluation of the teratogenicity of drugs.
         Clinical Pharmacology and Therapeutics, 1964, 5, 480-
         514.

1147.   Candeias, N. M. F. Fumo durante a gestacao: Aspectos
         educativos de um problema comportamental. (Smoking
         during pregnancy: Educational aspects of a behavior
         problem.) Revista de Saude Publica, 1979, 13, 244-253.

1148.   Cattanach, B. M. Lack of effect of nicotine on the fer-
         tility of male and female mice. Zeitschrift für Ver-
         erbungslehre, 1962, 93, 351-355.

1149.   Catz, C. S. and Giacoia, G. P. Drugs and breast milk.
         Pediatric Clinics of North America, 1972, 19, 151-166.

1150.   Cherry, L. Smoking: How real are the dangers for women?
         Glamour, 1979, 77, 250-251.

1150a.   Christianson, R. E. Relationship between maternal smoking
         and the incidence of congenital anomalies. American
         Journal of Epidemiology, 1980, 112, 684-695.

1151.   Chung, C. S. and Myrianthopoulos, N. C. Factors affecting
         risks of congenital malformations. I. Analysis of epi-
         demiologic factors in congenital malformations. Report
         from the Collaborative Perinatal project. Birth Defects:
         Original Article Series, 1975, 11, 1-19, 21-22.

1152.   Cooper, P. More thoughts for smoking mothers. Food and
         Cosmetics Toxicology, 1978, 16, 187-188.

1153.   Cooper, P. The smoking mother revisited. Food and Cos-
         metics Toxicology, 1978, 16, 187-188.

1153a.   Crosby, W. H., Metcoff, J., Costiloe, J. P., Mameesh, M.,
          Sandstead, H. H., Jacob, R. A., McClain, P. E.,
          Jacobson, G., Reid, W., and Burns, G. Fetal malnu-
          trition: An Appraisal of correlated factors. Amer-
          ican Journal of Obstetrics and Gynecology, 1977, 128,
          22-31.

D

1154.   Dalton, E. R., Hughes, C. A., and Cogswell, J. J.
         Cigarette smoking in pregnancy: A health education
         problem. Public Health, 1981, 95, 207-214.

1155.   Danaher, B. B. OB-GYN intervention in helping smokers
         quit. In Schwartz, J. L. (editor). Progress in
         Smoking Cessation. Proceedings of the International
         Conference on Smoking Cessation. New York, June 21-23,
         1978. American Cancer Society, 1979, 316-328.

1156.   Davies, D. P., Gray, O. P., Ellwood, P. C., and Aber-
         nethy, M. Cigarette smoking in pregnancy: Assoc-
         iations with maternal weight gain and fetal growth.
         Lancet, 1976, 1, 385-387.

1157.   Dawes, G. S. The physiological determinants of fetal
         growth. Journal of Reproduction and Fertility, 1976,
         47, 183-187.

1158.   Dayer, P. and Gross, G. Medicaments et grossesse.
         (Drugs and pregnancy.) Medicine et Hygiene, 1976, 34,
         427-428.

1159.   Dent, P. B., Chiavetta, J., Leeder, S., Richards, R., and
         Rawls, W. E. Elevated levels of carcinoembryonic
         antigen in cord plasma. Cancer, 1978, 42, 224-228.

1160.   Deshpande, T. V., Harding, P. G. R., and Jaco, N. T.
         Estimation of gestational age from study of amniotic
         fluid and clinical assessment. Canadian Medical As-
         sociation Journal, 1977, 117, 886-890.

1160a.   Drife, J. O. Drugs and sperm. British Medical Journal,
         1982, 284, 844.

1161.   D'Souza, S. W., Black, P., and Richards, B. Smoking in
         pregnancy: Associations with skinfold thickness,
         maternal weight gain, and fetal size at birth. British
         Medical Journal, 1981, 282, 1661-1663.

E

1162.   Edelson, E. Can drinking, smoking and pills
          harm your unborn baby? An update on the
          risks. Glamour, 1981, 79, 176.

1163.   Edwards, L. E., Alton, I. R., Barrada, M. I.,
          and Hakanson, E. Y. Pregnancy in the under-
          weight woman: Course, outcome, and growth
          patterns of the infant. American Journal of
          Obstetrics and Gynecology, 1979, 135, 297-302.

1164.   Eisinger, R. A. Cigarette smoking and the pedi-
          atrician: Findings based on a national
          survey. Clinical Pediatrics, 1972, 11, 645-
          647.

F

1165.   Fabia, J. Regression multiple du poids de naissance
         utilisant dix variables "predicatives." (Multiple
         regression of birth weight using ten predicative
         jariables.) Canadian Journal of Public Health, 1973,
         64, 548-551.

1166.   Fedrick, J. Antenatal identification of women at high
         risk of spontaneous pre-term birth. British Journal
         of Obstetrics and Gynecology, 1976, 83, 351-354.

1167.   Finnegan, L. P. In utero opiate dependence and sudden
         infant death syndrome. Clinics in Perinatology, 1979,
         6, 163-180.

1168.   Ford, B. Women and cigarettes: The deadly new evidence.
         Good Housekeeping, 1978, 187, 301-302.

1169.   Forrest, J. M. Drugs in pregnancy and lactation. Medical
         Journal of Australia, 1976, 2, 138-141.

1170.   Fraumeni, J. F. and Lundin, F. E. Smoking and pregnancy.
         Lancet, 1964, 1, 173.

G

1171. Galbraith, R. S., Karchmar, E. J., Piercy, W. N., and Low, J. A. The clinical prediction of intrauterine growth retardation. American Journal of Obstetrics and Gynecology, 1979, 133, 281-286.

1172. Garn, S. M. Tell pregnant patients: Do not smoke! Medical Times, 1980, 108, 18S-22S, 27S, 28S, 30S.

1173. Gavrilescu, C. Avortul spontan repetat. (Habitual spontaneous abortion.) Obstetrica si Ginecologia, 1973, 21, 201-208.

1174. Gelbart, S. M. and Sontag, S. J. Mutagenic urine in cirrhosis. Lancet, 1980, 1, 894-896.

1175. Geneja, M., Ilczyszyn, J., and Runge, T. Wpływ palenia papierosów na przebieg ciąży, termin porodu i stan noworodka bezpośrednio po porodzie. (Effect of smoking on pregnancy, labor, and the newborn.) Ginekologia Polska, 1979, Supplement, 66-68.

1176. Gennser, G., Marsal, K., and Brantmark, B. Maternal smoking and fetal breathing movements. American Journal of Obstetrics and Gynecology, 1975, 123, 861-867.

1177. Gianelli, A. and Scoppetta, V. Indagine comparativa sullo sviluppo ponderale dei nati da donne fumatrici e non fumatrici. (Comparative study of growth of newborns of smoking and nonsmoking mothers.) Arcispedale S. Anna di Ferrara, 1963, 16, 11-15.

1178. Gibel, W. and Blumberg, H. H. Die Auswirkungen der Rauchgewöhnheiten von Eltern auf das ungebornene und neugeborene Kind. (The effects of parental smoking habits on the unborn and newborn child.) Zeitschrift für Ärztliche Fortbildung, 1979, 73, 341-342.

1179.   Gibel, W. and Paun, D. Zu den Auswirkungen des Rauchens
         während der Schwangerschaft. (Effect of smoking on
         pregnancy.) In Givel, W. (editor). Gesundheitsschaden
         durch Rauchen--Möglichkeiten einer Prophylaxe. (Dam-
         ages to Health Through Smoking--Possibilities of a
         Preventive Measure.) Akademie-Verlag, Berlin, 1976,
         88-92.

1180.   Gofin, C. Smoking during pregnancy: A community survey.
         Journal of the Israel Medical Association, 1979, 96,
         278-281. (In Hebrew.)

1181.   Gordon, H. Gynaecology and obstetrics. Medical Annual,
         1972, 90, 204-216.

1182.   Gordon, Y. B., Lewis, J. D., Pendlebury, D. J., Leigh-
         ton, M., and Gold, J. Is measurement of placental
         function and maternal weight worthwhile? Lancet,
         1978, 1, 1001-1003.

1182a.   Gormican, A., Valentine, J., and Satter, E. Relation-
         ships of maternal weight gain, prepregnancy weight,
         and infant birthweight. Journal of the American
         Dietetic Association, 1980, 77, 662-667.

1183.   Gottsegen, J. J. Tobacco, A Study of Its Consumption in
         the United States. Pitman Publishing Company,
         New York, 1940.

1184.   Goujard, J., Hennequin, J. F., Kaminski, M., Marendas, R.,
         and Rumeau-Rouquette, C. Prevision de la prematurité
         et du poids de naissance en début de grossesse. (Pre-
         diction of prematurity and birthweight at the beginning
         of pregnancy.) Journal de Gynécologie Obstétrique et
         Biologie de la Reproduction, 1974, 3, 45-59.

1185.   Goujard, J., Kaminski, M., and Rumeau-Rouquette, C.
         Moyenne ponderale et âge gestationnel en relation avec
         quelques caracteristique maternelles. Enquête pros-
         pective portant sur une population d'enfants nès dans
         des maternités hospitalières de Paris. (Average weight
         and gestational age in relation to several maternal
         characteristics. Prospective study conducted on a
         population of infants born in maternity hospitals in
         Paris.) Archives Françaises de Pédiatrie, 1973, 30,
         341-362.

1186.   Grant, E. C. G. The harmful effects of common social
         habits, especially smoking and using oral contracep-
         tive steroids, on pregnancy. International Journal
         of Environmental Studies, 1981, 17, 57-66.

H

1187.   Halbe, H. W., Vieira, C., Gelas, G., Da Cunha, D. C., and
         Bagnoli, V. R.   Aspectos o ganho ponderal a gestante.
         (Aspects of weight gain in pregnancy.)   Jornal Brasil-
         eiro de Ginecologia, 1975, 80, 207-209.

1187a.   Hammer, R. E. and Mitchell, J. A.   Effects of nicotine
         on zona pellucida loss and blastocyst development in
         the rat.   Anatomical Record, 1979, 194, 629.

1188.   Hopkin, J. M. and Evans, H. J.   Cigarette smoke conden-
         sates damage DNA in human lymphocytes.   Nature, 1979,
         279, 241-242.

I

1189.   Illingsworth, R. S. Abnormal substances excreted in human milk. Practitioner, 1953, 171, 533-538.

J

1190.   Jensen, O. H. and Foss, O. P. Smoking in preg-
          nancy. Effect on the birth weight and on
          thiocyanate concentration in mother and baby.
          Acta Obstetrica et Gynecologica Scandinavica,
          1981, 60, 177-181.

1191.   Joffe, J. M. Influence of drug exposure of the
          father on perinatal outcome. Clinics in
          Perinatology, 1979, 6, 21-36.

1192.   Johnson, F. L., Winship, H. W., and Trinca, C. E.
          Neonatal medication surveillance by the
          pharmacist. American Journal of Hospital
          Pharmacy, 1977, 34, 609-612.

1193.   Johnson, J. W. C. and Dubin, N. H. Prevention
          of preterm labor. Clinical Obstetrics and
          Gynecology, 1980, 23, 51-73.

1194.   Johnstone, T. Primary prevention and low birth-
          weight. Lancet, 1982, 1, 805.

1195.   Junceda Avello, E. Factores medico-sociales en
          maternologia y su repercusion perinatologica.
          (Socio-medical factors in pregnancy and their
          perinatal consequences.) Toko-Ginecologia
          Practica, 1979, 38, 179-192.

K

1196.   Kagan, J. Special risks women smokers take. _McCalls_,
         1980, _107_, 57.

1197.   Karki, N. T., Pelkonen, O., Tuimala, R., Kauppila, A.,
         and Koivisto, M. Aryl hydrocarbon hydroxylase induc-
         tion in maternal and cord blood mitogen-treated lympho-
         cytes. _Developmental Pharmacology and Therapeutics_,
         1981, _2_, 32-43.

1198.   Kline, J., Shrout, P., Stein, Z., Susser, M., and War-
         burton, D. Drinking during pregnancy and spontaneous
         abortion. _Lancet_, 1980, _2_, 176-180.

1198a.   Klinge, E. Pharmacology and physiology of the bull re-
         tractor penis muscle. Fourth International Congress
         on Pharmacology, Basel, 1969 (abstract), 338-339.

1199.   Knowles, J. A. Excretion of drugs in milk--A review.
         Journal of Pediatrics, 1965, _66_, 1068-1082.

1200.   Kozak, J. and Novotna, M. Koureni tecotnych zen.
         (Smoking among pregnant women.) _Studia Pheumologica
         et Physiologica Cechoslovaca_, 1979, _39_, 364-368.

1201.   Kuhnert, P. M., Kuhnert, B. R., Bottoms, S. F., and
         Erhard, P. Cadmium levels in maternal blood, fetal
         cord blood, and placental tissues of pregnant women
         who smoke. _American Journal of Obstetrics and
         Gynecology_, 1982, _142_, 1021-1025.

1202.   Kulavskii, V. A. Kueniy i beremenmost. Obyor literatury.
         (Smoking and pregnancy. Review of the literature.)
         Akusherstvo i Ginekologiia, 1970, _46_, 68-70.

L

1203.   Laurenson, V. G. The effect of illegitimacy on the
         neonate. New Zealand Medical Journal, 1971, 74,
         377-381.

1204.   Lee, B. L. Women's drug/alcohol risks on rise.
         The Journal, 1979, August 1, 3.

1205.   Lee, B. L. Women smoking in labor are smoking for two.
         The Journal, 1979, August 1, 3.

1206.   Lehtovirta, P. Tupakointi ja raskaus. (Smoking and
         pregnancy.) Duodecim, 1979, 95, 5-7.

1207.   Lemberger, L. and Rubin, A. Physiologic Disposition of
         Drugs of Abuse. Spectrum Publications, New York, 1976.

1208.   Leon, L. High-risk pregnancy: Graphic representation
         of the maternal and fetal risks. American Journal of
         Obstetrics and Gynecology, 1973, 117, 497-504.

1209.   Lesigang, C. Neugeborenenneurologie und Entwicklungs-
         prognose. (New born neurology and developmental
         prognosis.) Paediatrie und Paedologie, 1974, 9,
         252-260.

1210.   Levin, R. H. Teratogenicity and drug excretion in
         breast milk (materogenicity). Clinical Pharmacology
         and Therapeutics, 1975, 16, 23-44.

1211.   Levine, K. What every pregnant woman needs to know.
         Redbook, 1980, 155, 56.

1212.   Linn, S., Schoenbaum, S. C., Monson, R. R., Rosner, B.,
         Stubblefield, P. G., and Ryan, K. J. No association
         between coffee consumption and adverse outcomes of
         pregnancy. New England Journal of Medicine, 1982,
         306, 141-145.

1213.   Low, J. A. Fetal breathing. Annals of the Royal College of Physicians and Surgeons of Canada, 1976, 9, 301-303.

1214.   Low, J.A., Galbraith, R. S., Muir, D., Killen, H., Karchmar, J., and Campbell, D. Intrauterine growth retardation: A preliminary report of long term morbidity. American Journal of Obstetrics and Gynecology, 1978, 130, 534-545.

1215.   Lubchenco, L. O. The infant who is small for gestational age. Major Problems in Clinical Pediatrics, 1976, 14, 181-201.

1216.   Luke, B., Hawkins, M. H., and Petrie, R. H. Influence of smoking, weight gain, and prepregnant weight for height on intrauterine growth. American Journal of Clinical Nutrition, 1981, 34, 1410-1417.

M

1217.   Mackie, A. Women and smoking. In Steinfeld, J., Grif-
         fiths, W., Ball, K., and Taylor, R. M. (editors).
         Public Health Service: Health Consequences, Educa-
         tion, Cessation Activities, and Governmental Action.
         U. S. Department of Health, Education, and Welfare,
         DHEW Publication No. (NIH) 77-1413, 1975, pp. 403-
         407.

1218.   Majewski, A. Obraz kliniczny zatru ia nikotyna noworod-
         kow karmionych piersia. (Clinical manifestations of
         nicotine intoxication in breast-fed infants.) Wiado-
         mosci Lekarskie, 1979, 32, 275-277.

1219.   Majewski, F. Über einige durch teratogene Noxen indu-
         zierte Fehlbildungen. (On certain embryopathies
         produced by teratogens.) Monatsschrift für Kinder-
         heilkunde, 1977, 125, 609-620.

1219a.   Malinas, Y. Hygiene de la grossesse. (Health care in
         pregnancy.) Concours Medical, 1974, 96 (Supplement
         16), 45-48.

1220.   Manning, F. A. Fetal breathing movements as a reflec-
         tion of fetal status. Postgraduate Medicine, 1977,
         61, 116-122.

1220a.   Manning, M. D. and Carroll, B. E. Some epidemiological
         aspects of leukemia in children. Journal of the
         National Cancer Institute, 1957, 19, 1087-1094.

1221.   Martin, J. C. and Becker, R. F. The effects of nicotine
         administration in utero upon activity in the rat.
         Psychonomic Science, 1970, 19, 59-60.

1221a.   Murthy, P. B. K. Frequency of sister chromatid ex-
         changes in cigarette smokers. Human Genetics, 1979,
         52, 343-345.

N

1222.   Nicolicchia, M.-A. <u>Uso, ed Abuso del Tabacco</u>. (<u>Use and Abuse of Tobacco</u>.) Lyons, 1708.

O

1223.   O'Brien, T. E. Excretion of drugs in human milk.
        American Journal of Hospital Pharmacy, 1974, 31,
        844-854.

P

1224.   Papoz, L., Eschwege, E., Pequignot, G., Barrat, J., and
        Schwartz, D. Maternal smoking and birth weight in
        relation to dietary habits. American Journal of Ob-
        stetrics and Gynecology, 1982, 142, 870-876.

1225.   Pettersson, F., Fries, H., and Nillius, S. Epidemiology
        of secondary amenorrhea. I. Incidence and prevalence
        rates. American Journal of Obstetrics and Gynecology,
        1973, 117, 80-86.

1225a. Primrose, T. and Higgins, A. A study in human antepartum
        birth weight nutrition. Journal of Reproductive
        Medicine, 1971, 7, 257-264.

R

1226.　　Rich, B.　The Honestie of This Age.　London, 1615.

S

1227.   Schrauzer, G. N., Rhead, W. J., and Saltzstein, S. L.
         Sudden infant death syndrome: Plasma vitamin E levels
         and dietary factors. Annals of Clinical and Laboratory
         Science, 1975, 5, 31-37.

T

1228.   Thoa, N. B. and Maengwyn-Davies, G. D. The guinea-pig
         isolated vas deferens: A method for increasing
         sensitivity to drugs. Journal of Pharmaceutics and
         Pharmacology, 1968, 20, 873-876.

V

1229.   Vaughan, W. <u>Directions</u> <u>for</u> Health, Naturall and Arti-
         ficiall: <u>Derived</u> <u>from</u> <u>the</u> <u>best</u> Phisitians, as <u>well</u>
         Moderne as Antient. <u>Divided</u> <u>into</u> 6 Sections <u>compre</u>
         hending 1. <u>Ayre</u>, <u>Fire</u>, and Water. 2. Foode <u>and</u>
         <u>Nourishment</u>. 3. <u>Evacuations</u>, <u>as</u> Purgations, Tobacco-
         <u>taking</u>, &c. 4. <u>Infirmities</u>, <u>Humours</u>, and Death.
         5. <u>Perturbations</u> of the <u>mind</u>, and <u>spirituall</u> sick-
         <u>nesses</u>. 6. <u>Quarterly</u>, <u>Monethly</u>, and <u>Daily</u> Diet, with
         <u>Medicines</u> to <u>prolong</u> <u>life</u>. Sixth edition. John Beale,
         London, 1626.

1229a.   Vessey, M. P., Wright, N. H., McPherson, K., and Wig-
         gins, P. Fertility after stopping different methods
         of contraception. British <u>Medical</u> <u>Journal</u>, 1978, <u>1</u>,
         265-267.

1230.   Viczián, M. and Heinisch, P. A dohanyzas hatasa a
         spermatogenesisre. (The effects of smoking on
         spermatogenesis.) <u>Magyar</u> <u>Noorvosok</u> <u>Lapja</u>, 1967, <u>35</u>,
         412-418.

1230a.   Villumsen, A. L. Environmental factors in congenital
         malformations: A prospective study of 9,006 human
         pregnancies. Diss. published by F.A.D.L., Copenhagen-
         Arhus-Odense, 1970.

W

1231. Wigle, D. T., Mao, Y., and Grace, M. Smoking and cancer of the uterine cervix: Hypothesis. *American Journal of Epidemiology*, 1980, 111, 125-127.

Y

1232.   Yun, I. S. and Lee, Y. S. Experimental studies on the
         relation between nicotine and sexual hormone.
         Folia Endocrinology Japan, 1935, 11, 9-12.

Index